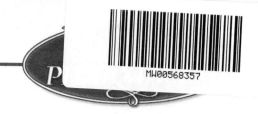

Inside—Find the Answers to These Questions and More

☑ What is black cohosh, and can it help relieve my menopausal symptoms? (See page 66.)

☑ Can I take black cohosh even if I had breast cancer? (See page 76.)

☑ Can the supplement ipriflavone prevent and treat osteoporosis? (See page 103.)

☑ How does ipriflavone compare with standard treatments for osteoporosis? (See page 104.)

☑ Why should I take calcium and how can it help osteoporosis? (See page 110.)

☑ Can the herb kava help anxiety related to menopause? (See page 78.)

☑ What are the benefits of soy for menopause? (See page 97.)

☑ How can I reduce my risk of cardiovascular disease after menopause? (See page 27.)

☑ What is "natural" progesterone? (See page 13.)

☑ What are the benefits and risks of hormone-replacement therapy? (See page 34.)

THE NATURAL PHARMACIST Library

Arthritis

Diabetes

Echinacea and Immunity

Feverfew and Migraines

Garlic and Cholesterol

Ginkgo and Memory

Heart Disease Prevention

Herbs

Illnesses and Their Natural Remedies

Kava and Anxiety

Menopause

PMS

Reducing Cancer Risk

Saw Palmetto and the Prostate

St. John's Wort and Depression

Vitamins and Supplements

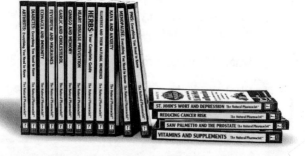

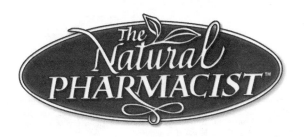

Everything You Need to Know About

Menopause

Joanne Marie Snow

Series Editors

Steven Bratman, M.D.

David Kroll, Ph.D.

A DIVISION OF PRIMA PUBLISHING

Visit us online at www.thenaturalpharmacist.com

Warning—Disclaimer

Library of Congress Cataloging-in-Publication Data

Snow, Joanne Marie.
    Menopause / Joanne Marie Snow.
        p.   cm.—(The natural pharmacist)
    Includes bibliographical references and index.
    ISBN 0-7615-1560-7
    1. Menopause—Popular works.   I. Title.   II. Series.
RG186.S696 1999
612.6'65—dc21   98—38774
                                                                      CIP

00 01 02 HH 10 9 8 7 6 5 4 3
Printed in the United States of America

Visit us online at www.thenaturalpharmacist.com

Contents

Contents

What Makes This Book Different?

The interest in natural medicine has never been greater. According to the National Association of Chain Drug Stores, 65 million Americans are using natural supplements, and the number is growing! Yet it is hard for the consumer to find trustworthy sources for balanced information about this emerging field. Why? Frankly, natural medicine has had a checkered history. From snake oil potions sold at the turn of the century to those books, magazines, and product catalogs that hype miracle cures today, this is a field where exaggerated claims have been the norm. Proponents of natural medicine have tended to abuse science, treating it more as a marketing tool than a means of discovering the truth.

But there is truth to be found. Studies of vitamins, minerals, and other food supplements have been with us since these nutritional substances were first discovered, and the level and quality of this science has grown dramatically in the last 20 years. Herbal medicine has been neglected in the United States, but in Europe, this, the oldest of all healing arts, has been the subject of tremendous and ongoing scientific interest.

At present, for a number of herbs and supplements, it is possible to give reasonably scientific answers to the questions: How well does this work? How safe is it? What types of conditions is it best used for?

THE NATURAL PHARMACIST series is designed to cut through the hype and tell you what we know and what we don't know about popular natural treatments. These books are more conservative than any others available, more honest about the weaknesses of natural approaches, more fair in their comparisons of natural and conventional treatments. You won't find any miracle cures here, but you will discover useful options that can help you become healthier.

Why Choose Natural Treatments?

Although the science behind natural medicine continues to grow, this is still a much less scientifically validated field than conventional medicine. You might ask, "Why should I resort to an herb that is only partly proven, when I could take a drug with solid science behind it?" There are at least three good reasons to consider natural alternatives.

First, some herbs and supplements offer benefits that are not matched by any conventional drug. Vitamin E is a good example. It appears to help prevent prostate cancer, a benefit that no standard medication can claim. Also, vitamin E almost certainly helps prevent heart disease. While there are standard drugs that also prevent heart disease, vitamin E works differently and may be able to complement many of the other approaches.

Another example is the herb milk thistle. Studies strongly suggest that this herb can protect the liver from injury. There is no pill or tablet your doctor can prescribe to do the same.

Even if the science behind some of these treatments is less than perfect, when the risks are low and the possible benefit high, a treatment may be worth trying. It is a little-known fact that for many conventional treatments the science is less than perfect as well, and physicians must balance uncertain benefits against incompletely understood risks.

A second reason to consider natural therapies is that some may offer benefits comparable to those of drugs with fewer side effects. The herb St. John's wort is a good example. Reasonably strong scientific evidence suggests that this herb is an effective treatment for mild to moderate depression, while producing fewer side effects on average than conventional medications. Saw palmetto for benign enlargement of the prostate, ginkgo for relieving symptoms and perhaps slowing the progression of Alzheimer's disease, and glucosamine for osteoarthritis are other examples. This is not to say that herbs and supplements are completely harmless—they're not—but for most the level of risk is quite low.

Finally, there is a philosophical point to consider. For many people, it "feels" better to use a treatment that comes from nature instead of from a laboratory. Just as you might rather wear all-cotton clothing than polyester, or look at a mountain landscape rather than the skyscrapers of a downtown city, natural treatments may simply feel more compatible with your view of life. We can quibble endlessly about just what "natural" means and whether a certain treatment is "actually" natural or not, but such arguments are beside the point. The difference is in the feeling, and feelings matter. In fact, having a good feeling about taking an herb may lead you to use it more consistently than you would a prescription drug.

Of course, at times synthetic drugs may be necessary and even lifesaving. But on many other occasions it may be quite reasonable to turn to an herb or supplement instead of a drug.

To make good decisions you need good information. Unfortunately, while hundreds of books on alternative medicine are published every year, many are highly misleading. The phrase "studies prove" is often used when the studies in question are so small or so badly conducted that they prove nothing at all. You may even find that the "data" from other books comes from studies with petri dishes and not real people!

You can't even assume that books written by well-known authors are scientifically sound. Many of these authors rely on secondary writers, leading to a game of "telephone," where misconceptions are passed around from book to book. And there's a strong tendency to exaggerate the power of natural remedies, whitewashing them with selective reporting.

THE NATURAL PHARMACIST series gives you the balanced information you need to make informed decisions about your health needs. Setting a new, high standard of accuracy and objectivity, these books take a realistic look at the herbs and supplements you read about in the news. You will encounter both favorable and unfavorable studies in these pages and will learn about both the benefits and the risks of natural treatments.

THE NATURAL PHARMACIST series is the source you can trust.

Steven Bratman, M.D.
David Kroll, Ph.D.

Introduction

It is estimated that there are 20 million women in the United States presently in menopause. By the year 2010 the number will increase to 60 million. Worldwide, approximately 24.5 million women reach menopause each year.

These statistics are impressive. If you are in or approaching menopause, you are certainly not alone. However, many women feel frustrated and confused. I've talked to hundreds of women who feel lost in a sea of conflicting information.

There is no way to know in advance how one is going to experience menopause. Each woman experiences menopause differently from the next woman. There are some women who have physical symptoms such as hot flashes, and other women who experience no physical symptoms whatsoever.

Today, through the advances of science, we have a better understanding of what happens in the body during menopause. We now understand that the natural decline of hormone levels that occurs throughout menopause is responsible for numerous physical symptoms, such as hot flashes, and may also lead to osteoporosis and heart disease.

Science has developed hormone therapies in an attempt to supplement this natural decline, with the hopes of alleviating the suffering of many women. Many women question, is this natural? We know that hormone-replacement therapy does help, but there are also risks involved with this type of treatment.

There are so many questions that women want answered: What is happening in my body? Why do I feel so different? What are the benefits and risks of hormone-replacement therapy? Are there more "natural" methods to help with symptoms? Are there foods that I can eat that will help my body? What other types of therapies are available? What can I do to help protect against osteoporosis and heart disease? *The Natural Pharmacist Guide to Menopause* will answer these questions and will provide an awareness into how to ease into this transitional period in your life.

Chapter 1 will discuss what happens to your body during menopause, from the ebb and flow of hormone levels, to the physical "symptoms" which may result from this change.

Chapter 2 will address the health risks of osteoporosis and cardiovascular disease, which are associated with menopause, and will focus on what you can do to reduce your risk of developing these conditions. Chapter 3 is dedicated to hormone-replacement therapy, where the facts, both pros and cons, are presented for your evaluation.

Chapters 4 through 9 are dedicated to natural remedies and lifestyle changes that can significantly reduce menopause-related symptoms and help protect against cardiovascular disease and osteoporosis.

Chapters 4 through 7 will discuss herbs, such as black cohosh, that have been clinically shown to significantly reduce menopausal symptoms. Chapter 8 will examine phytoestrogens: what they are, how we believe they work, and how they might help your body. Chapter 9 discusses supplements such as vitamins, minerals, and essential fatty acids that can also reduce menopausal symptoms and protect against heart disease and osteoporosis.

Chapter 10 will focus on lifestyle changes such as exercise and stress reduction, which can help to maintain health and well-being during menopause. The last chapter discusses alternative therapies that have shown to be very effective in treating menopausal symptoms.

The Natural Pharmacist Guide to Menopause seeks to empower you, the wonderful woman that you are, to make informed choices in how you wish to assist or to not assist your body in the transition we call menopause.

What Is Menopause?

When I first spoke with Sarah, she wanted help for her insomnia. Always a heavy sleeper, she had suddenly begun to have trouble falling asleep at night. I asked her if she had noticed any other physical changes. She mentioned strange new fluctuations in her menstrual cycle, stating that her flow might not come for 45 or 50 days, and when it did, it was sometimes unusually heavy. Then one day while standing in line at the grocery store, she broke out in a heavy sweat. Her hot flash confirmed my suspicion that Sarah was entering menopause.

Menopause is the end of a woman's childbearing years, marked by the end of menstruation. It is a natural change that generally happens in a woman's late 40s or early 50s. Doctors consider a woman to be in menopause when she's gone 12 consecutive months without a menstrual period. This change is a result of the body's natural decrease in the production of sex hormones. These hormonal changes can produce symptoms that range from subtle to very intense.

Although hot flashes are the most common menopausal symptom, Sarah's story shows that other symptoms can come first. For some women, emotional changes are the first sign of menopause. Anne is a good example.

Anne called me one day, very upset. I could hear the tension in her voice. She explained, "I don't know myself anymore. It's not just mood swings; it feels like I'm having radical changes in my personality from day to day. I've never been like this before, and I don't know what to do with myself."

Anne was also experiencing the first signs of menopause. Like many women, at first she didn't know what was happening to her body, and it scared her. "If I knew why it was happening," she said, "I would be less afraid. I just want to understand."

In this chapter, I will explain what menopause is, what causes it, and the symptoms you can expect. In later chapters I will explore all of your options to make this natural transition more graceful.

Types of Menopause

Technically, the term *menopause* indicates the last episode of menstrual bleeding in a woman's life. However, the term is often used more broadly to indicate the entire duration of time measured from when periods first become irregular up to the end of hot flashes and other symptoms. (The scientific term for this long interval is *climacteric*.)

Menopause can be natural or artificial. *Natural menopause* typically occurs between the ages of 49 and 51, but it can happen at any time during a woman's 40s or 50s, and some women experience menopause as early as their 30s. Natural menopause occurs when the ovaries can no longer produce viable ova (eggs). The result is a dramatic fall in levels of estrogen and progesterone, as well as other hormones such as androstenedione and testosterone (yes, women have testosterone, too!). Genetics play an important part in determining the age at which your natural menopause will begin. Although we're not sure exactly how, factors such as cigarette smoking also appear to influence the onset of natural menopause. Autoimmune diseases and other conditions can cause menopause to occur prematurely.[1]

Natural menopause typically occurs between the ages of 49 and 51, but it can happen at any time during a woman's 40s or 50s.

The other kind of menopause is called *artificial* (or *sudden*) *menopause* and, as the name suggests, it is created artificially—for example, by the surgical removal of both ovaries. Artificial menopause can also occur when the ovaries are damaged by radiation, chemotherapy, or various other drug therapies. Unlike natural menopause, which gives you a chance to get used to your hormones gradually fading away, with sudden menopause the production of these hormones comes to a screeching halt. The symptoms of menopause appear overnight.

For example, when my friend Amy took the drug Lupron for endometriosis, she suddenly began to experience intense hot flashes. "With no warning, I would go into a full dripping sweat," Amy said. "I didn't know what hit me." Lupron had radically reduced her body's hormone levels, throwing her into instant menopause.

Artificial menopause presents an even greater challenge than natural menopause, because it arrives so quickly. With natural menopause, you have time to adjust to what is happening, both physically and emotionally. But your response will depend to a great deal on your attitude toward it. Do

you view it as a disease or as a natural transition? The
answer may depend on what part of the world you live in
and whose evaluation of menopause you rely on.

Medical and Cultural Views of Menopause

Since the 1960s, the medical profession has viewed menopause as an estrogen-deficiency disease, a condition that
should be treated and managed. This viewpoint is ex-
pressed in medical texts, where menopausal women's bodies are commonly described in terms of "decline" or
"failed production." Women's breasts and ovaries are said
to "atrophy," "wither," and become "senile."[2] According to
a pivotal book on the subject, women become "female eu-
nuchs." Hormone-replacement therapy (HRT) is viewed
as a treatment for the "disease" of menopause.

The notion of menopause as a "disease" is not much
different from the view held during the nineteenth century, when it was commonly believed that menopause
could cause insanity. Victorian-era court records indicate
that "moral insanity" due to menopause was often accepted as a defense in cases of shoplifting.[3]

Today, our beliefs about menopause are influenced by
the way our society views old age. Advertisements,
movies, and TV perpetuate the idea that we are only of
value to society if we remain forever young. We are taught
that old age is something to fear rather than to embrace.
We worry that we will become incontinent, fatigued, for-
getful, senile, and irrelevant to the world as it marches on.

Despite these pervasive attitudes, my grandmother
Cecile had a positive attitude about aging. She was healthy
and lived independently until the age of 94. She would
laugh and say, "You're as old as you feel," and she knew
the importance of physical fitness and the need to keep
moving. In fact, I remember her storing things in her cab-

inets just out of reach so that she would have to stretch to retrieve them. She kept up her busy lifestyle until only a few months before her death.

The herbalist Susun Weed shares my grandmother's positive view of aging. She describes menopause as a metamorphosis, as "the years of transformation from potential mother to wise, whole crone."[4] This approach has been sometimes called the Wise Woman tradition, a belief that wisdom comes with age and that women past menopause should be respected. In this movement, the word *crone* is taken as a compliment rather than an insult, a recognition of the value and power of age.

In Western society, this attitude may sound alien and unacceptable to many women. But in Japan, most women believe that *konenki*—menopause—is a natural transition.[5] This attitude of acceptance may even affect the symptoms of menopause. In a survey of 1,316 women in Japan, anthropologist Margaret Lock found that only 9.7% had hot flashes and 3.5% experienced night sweats. The most common complaint (52%) was stiff shoulders.[6] Dr. Lock also interviewed 30 Japanese doctors, who confirmed her findings. The doctors reported that the most common symptoms menopausal women experienced were shoulder stiffness, headaches, and dizziness. There is no word in Japanese for "hot flash," but the closest equivalent words for this symptom ranked at the bottom of the list.

Dr. Lock's findings are supported by another cross-cultural study conducted in Chichimila, Mexico. In this study, Mayan women reported that they neither experienced hot flashes nor recalled other significant menopausal symptoms. The Mayan culture views menopause as a positive event, not as something to fear.[7] In the United States, where the cultural view of menopause is more negative than positive, some physicians report that 80 to 90% of menopausal women experience hot flashes.[8]

Commonly Used Terms

There are so many words used to describe menopause. Here are definitions of some of the most common.

Menopause: Technically, the final episode of menstrual bleeding, but the term is sometimes used synonymously with *climacteric.*

Climacteric: The period of declining female hormones, beginning in a woman's 40s, and often continuing into her 70s.

Premenopause: The time prior to menopause.

Perimenopause: The time just before and after menopause, when hot flashes and other immediate symptoms of menopause develop.

Postmenopause: Technically, the time after the last episode of menstrual bleeding, but the term is often used to indicate the time when perimenopausal symptoms stop and more long-term changes set in.

Of course, it's hard to tell which came first—positive attitude or fewer symptoms. Perhaps the soybeans that are so prevalent in the Japanese diet (and unknown factors in the Mayan diet) counteract menopausal symptoms (see chapter 8 for more information on the use of soy products to treat the symptoms of menopause). Thus women may have a positive attitude toward menopause because their symptoms are mild, rather than the reverse. Still, if Western culture had a more positive view about aging to begin with, perhaps we would experience fewer unpleasant menopausal symptoms. Maybe we could even enjoy the transition of menopause.

The Physical and Emotional Changes of Menopause

As Sarah and Anne can tell you, most women experience menopause as a process, not as a single event. During the months or years leading up to menopause and for some time after—a period technically known as *perimenopause* (meaning "around the time of menopause")—a woman experiences a gradual transition as her hormone levels slowly decrease and her body undergoes many physical and emotional changes. The good news about perimenopause is that its symptoms, however uncomfortable, are temporary. The body eventually adjusts to the new levels of estrogen, progesterone, and other hormones, and these symptoms disappear. From that point on, a woman is said to be "postmenopausal." Hot flashes are replaced by other effects of permanently lowered hormone levels (unless she takes hormones or other treatments with hormonal effects).

The good news about perimenopause is that its symptoms, however uncomfortable, are temporary.

I have been referring to the physical and emotional changes experienced during menopause as *symptoms*. Because they are natural, it would be better to call them "normal changes," or just "experiences." However, since they are ordinarily referred to as symptoms, I will do so here, though with considerable reluctance!

Symptoms of Perimenopause

The most common symptoms of the perimenopausal period are menstrual irregularity, hot flashes, and mood swings.

Menstrual Irregularity

Hormonal fluctuations during perimenopause can cause irregular menstrual cycles for 1 to 5 years before actual menopause. Your cycle may lengthen and you may skip some periods altogether. Other women have very erratic cycles: 18 to 20 days followed by 60 days or longer.

Besides the fluctuation in cycle length, some women experience heavy bleeding, either as a rapid flow or as a more moderate flow over a longer period of time. The level of bleeding often fluctuates as well—a woman might have a heavy flow one month and a light flow the next.

Profuse bleeding can be accompanied by large blood clots, which can be painful to pass and may leave a woman feeling weak and tired. Heavy menstrual bleeding can be an uncomfortable and frightening experience. If the bleeding is prolonged or frequent, you can lose enough blood to become anemic.

It is always recommended that you consult your doctor if your period becomes irregular, because this can also be a sign of uterine cancer.

As we will discuss further in chapter 3, progesterone is sometimes used to help excessive bleeding.

Hot Flashes

Hot flashes usually come on without warning. All of a sudden, you start to feel strange. Your face and neck become hot and sweat breaks out on your forehead, the back of your neck, or perhaps all over your body. Your heart starts to race and you may grab something to fan yourself with— but before you know it, the hot flash fades away.

My friend Cara experiences an average of one or two hot flashes each day. She reports that they aren't too bad, but they *can* be inconvenient. For relief from her hot flashes, she keeps a small, portable mini-fan in her pocketbook and uses it when she needs to.

Hot flashes are the most common menopausal symptom among Western women. Eighty percent of menopausal American women experience hot flashes, and almost 40% consider them enough of a problem to seek medical help.[9]

Hot flashes can last from 30 seconds to 5 minutes. Some women have only a few a year, while others may experience one or more per day. Some women, like Cara, sweat very little with their hot flashes, but others sweat profusely. Some women only experience hot flashes during the day, while others may be

There are many natural treatments that seem to stop hot flashes.

awakened at night. One woman said, "I dream that I'm in a hot shower and can't get out. Then I wake up and realize it's a hot flash."

Hot flashes can be triggered by stress, caffeine, and alcohol, and they also occur in people who are not menopausal. We don't know exactly what causes hot flashes, but estrogen is clearly involved, because treatment with estrogen stops hot flashes. Also, thin women tend to have more severe and frequent hot flashes than women who are heavier, and fat cells are known to make estrogen.[10]

As we'll see in chapter 5 and chapters 7 through 11 there are many natural treatments that seem to stop hot flashes. The one with the best evidence behind it is black cohosh, but soy products and many other options may be helpful as well.

Mood Swings

Not all women experience mood swings during menopause, but for those who do, these hormonally induced states of

Fluctuations in Hormone Levels

The following conditions may result when hormone levels rise and/or fall:

Irregular menstruation	Hot flashes
Mood swings	Fuzzy thinking
Night sweats	Insomnia
Thinning of body hair	Increase in facial hair
Lightheadedness	Dizzy spells
Fluctuations in sexual desire	Weight gain
Memory problems	Fluid retention

irritability, anxiety, or depression can be quite intense. Some women report that they're similar to the mood variations that are experienced during premenstrual syndrome (PMS).

The causes of mood swings are complex and not fully understood. We do know that estrogen and progesterone—the two most important sex hormones involved in menopause—have a profound effect on our emotions. Estrogen appears to act as a stimulant in the body: When a woman's estrogen levels are high, she may experience anxiety and irritability. Progesterone is believed to have a sedative effect: When a woman's progesterone levels are high, she may experience fatigue and depression.[11] As you'll see in chapters 5, 6, and 10, menopausal mood swings may respond well to natural treatments such as black cohosh, kava, and lifestyle changes.

Other Symptoms of Perimenopause

Fluctuations in hormone levels during perimenopause may also cause fuzzy thinking, night sweats, insomnia, thinning of body hair, increase in facial hair, lightheadedness, dizzy spells, fluctuations in sexual desire, weight gain, memory problems, and fluid retention.

Symptoms of Postmenopause

Once your menstruation has stopped and the rapid fluctuations in your natural hormone levels have been replaced by a slow and gradual decline, postmenopause brings a different set of changes in your body. These symptoms or changes tend to be more long-term. Hormone-replacement therapy as well as several natural therapies can help alleviate or reduce these symptoms.

Vaginal Dryness

One of the most distressing symptoms of postmenopause is vaginal dryness, which can cause itching and make sexual intercourse painful. When estrogen levels dwindle, as they do during peri- and postmenopause, blood flow to the genital area decreases and the vaginal and urethral linings become thinner and less well-lubricated. The acidity of a woman's vagina may change as well, leaving her more vulnerable to infections. Vaginal dryness can occur during perimenopause as well as during postmenopause.[12]

The simplest remedy for vaginal dryness is a lubricant such as KY-Jelly. Some women prefer to use cold-pressed castor oil or vitamin E oil. Hormone-replacement therapy dramatically reduces symptoms of vaginal dryness, and certain alternative therapies such as black cohosh may be helpful as well (see chapter 5).

Other Symptoms of Postmenopause

During the postmenopausal years, some women develop additional symptoms, which can include bladder disturbances such as stress incontinence, skin wrinkling, facial hair growth, and loss of sexual desire. In addition, as we'll see in chapter 2, there is an increased risk of heart disease and osteoporosis.

What Causes Menopausal Symptoms?

The fluctuations and decreases in hormone levels that occur during the menopausal period are undoubtedly the cause of menopausal symptoms. However, this is a very complex subject and one that isn't fully understood.

This section will give a brief overview of what we know. If you prefer, you can skip ahead to read the chapters on treatment. However, the explanations I will give later in the book, about the way various treatments work, depend on your understanding the hormone changes that cause menopause. These hormonal changes are described in the following sections.

What Are Hormones?

Hormones are chemicals that act as messengers in the body, traveling through the bloodstream to trigger specific responses in other parts of the body.

There are many different kinds of hormones. Some directly act on organs, others target glands and cause them to produce other hormones, and some do both. Estrogen and progesterone are the two most important hormones involved in the female reproductive system and in menopause.

Estrogen

Technically, the right term is *estrogens,* not *estrogen,* because there are many hormones in the estrogen family. They are all linked together by their capacity to promote development of the uterine wall and other tissues such as the breasts. There are three primary estrogens found in the bloodstream:

- Estradiol
- Estrone
- Estriol

The ovaries produce estradiol and a smaller amount of estrone. Both estradiol and estrone are converted by the body into estriol.

To make this less confusing, from here on I'll refer to each of these three separate estrogens as simply *estrogen*, except when I specifically want to discuss a particular one.

Scientists have yet to discover the full range of estrogen's effects in the body. Besides affecting a woman's reproductive system, estrogen decreases the rate of bone reabsorption. As you'll see in chapter 2, this is a good thing: the less estrogen in your body, the faster the rate of bone reabsorption and the more likely you are to develop osteoporosis. Estrogen also helps prevent atherosclerosis, or hardening of the arteries, which causes heart disease and strokes. (For more information, see chapter 2.)

Estrogen also affects numerous other parts of your body. Estrogen that is not matched (technically, "opposed") by a proper amount of progesterone increases your risk of uterine cancer and probably also of breast cancer.

In menopause, levels of all the estrogens decrease, leading to vaginal thinning and dryness, changes in the bladder, an increased risk of osteoporosis and heart disease, and many other symptoms. As we shall see in later chapters, substances called *phytoestrogens*, which are found in foods, may be able to counteract some of the problems caused by reduced estrogen levels.

Progesterone

Progesterone gets its name from its ability to promote pregnancy (gestation). It is released during the second half of the menstrual cycle (after ovulation) and also throughout pregnancy. Progesterone produces numerous changes in the uterus and breasts, but we don't fully understand its effects on the rest of the body. We also don't understand how the decrease in progesterone levels that occurs during menopause affects the body.

The "progesterone" that is most commonly prescribed as a part of birth control pills or for other uses is not really progesterone; it's actually one of a couple of chemical cousins known as progestins. True progesterone is sometimes called "natural progesterone," and, as we will discuss in chapter 3, it may be helpful in relieving menopausal symptoms such as hot flashes.

Hormone Production in the Menstrual Cycle

To understand the changes that menopause brings, we must first review the normal menstrual cycle. Each month, estrogen is secreted by the ovaries and it signals the uterine lining to grow. After ovulation, progesterone causes significant swelling of the uterine lining to create a rich, blood-filled cushion, ready and waiting to nourish a fertilized egg. If conception does not occur, the uterus cleanses itself by releasing the extra blood and tissue—the *endometrium*—so that the cycle can begin anew. That's menstruation.

The mechanism that regulates the buildup and shedding of uterine lining is controlled by fluctuations in hormone levels. These fluctuations are based on complicated interactions between two organs that oversee most of the hormones in the body: the pituitary gland and the hypothalamus (see figure 1). The hypothalamus releases chemicals into the bloodstream to stimulate the pituitary gland. Based on this signal as well as others that it receives directly from the body, the pituitary gland releases follicle-stimulating hormone (FSH) and luteinizing hormone (LH). These hormones in turn control the ovaries.

The ovaries are two small, almond-shaped glands located in the pelvis on either side of the uterus. When you're born, your ovaries contain all the eggs you'll have

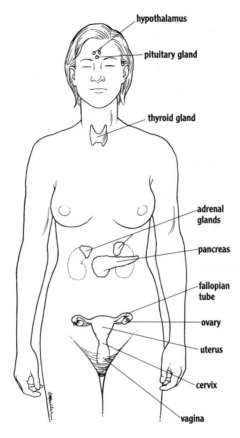

Figure 1. *Female reproductive anatomy*

throughout your lifetime. The eggs are in a dormant form called a *follicle*. At birth, each woman may have as many as one million follicles; by puberty that number drops to about 300,000 to 400,000. The follicles continue to decrease in number throughout a woman's life.

Each month, FSH and LH from the pituitary gland stimulate the follicles to produce estrogen. Some of them begin to enlarge, and eventually one of them ruptures, releasing an ovum. This is ovulation.

At birth, each woman may have as many as one million follicles; by puberty, that number drops to about 300,000 to 400,000. The follicles continue to decrease in number throughout a woman's lifetime.

Once it has released the ovum, the remaining part of the follicle further enlarges and becomes a structure called the corpus luteum (see figure 2). It produces progesterone and estrogen in preparation for pregnancy.

If the ovum is not fertilized, the corpus luteum soon deteriorates and hormone levels drop. Menstruation is the result: The lining of the uterus deteriorates and sloughs off, producing the familiar monthly bleeding.

Hormone Production in Menopause

By the time most women reach their early 40s, they have ovulated regularly for almost 30 years. During this time, the number of follicles (dormant eggs) in the ovaries has diminished, and the remaining follicles now produce less estrogen.

In the transition to menopause, ovulation occurs with decreasing frequency. Cycles begin to occur in which no follicles mature enough to release an ovum. Progesterone production is limited because without ovulation there is no corpus luteum to secrete progesterone. When progesterone and estrogen levels are low, the pituitary tries to compensate by increasing the levels of FSH and LH. At first this manages to stimulate hormone levels to some extent, but not reliably. This phase leads to the irregular pe-

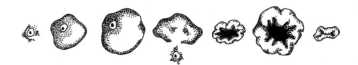

Figure 2. *Ovarian cycle*

riods of early perimenopause. Eventually your periods stop as the follicles give up altogether. Sky-high FHS and LH levels, due to the pituitary's vain attempts to raise estrogen and progesterone levels, are an objective sign that menopause has occurred (see table 1).

Once the ovaries stop producing ova, the adrenal glands take over hormone production. However, the adrenal glands can't produce enough hormones to restore premenopausal levels.

Women experience this decline in hormone levels in different ways. Some woman simply stop having their periods and have no symptoms whatsoever. Other women endure intense physical and emotional changes.

All treatments for menopause seek to restore hormonal balance or alleviate the symptoms caused by reduced hormone levels. Hormone-replacement therapy

Table 1. Hormonal levels

Phase	FSH (IU/liter)	LH (IU/liter)	*Estradiol (pmol/liter)
Premenopausal	2–10	5–25	100–600
Postmenopausal	40–70	50–70	60

*Estradiol is the primary form of estrogen.

(HRT) is the treatment preferred by most physicians. The pros and cons of HRT are discussed in chapter 3.

Natural remedies such as soy, black cohosh, various dietary supplements, and lifestyle changes can directly affect hormone levels or make up for reduced levels of hormones in other ways. Compared to HRT, these treatments have both pros and cons. They will be discussed in greater detail in chapter 5 and chapters 8 through 10.

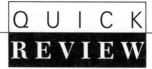

QUICK REVIEW

- Menopause is a natural change that marks the end of menstruation and, therefore, the end of childbearing years.

- During perimenopause and postmenopause, women may experience various physical and emotional changes, or "symptoms," that are caused by fluctuations in hormone levels.

- Fluctuations of estrogen levels cause the majority of menopause-related symptoms. These can include menstrual irregularity, hot flashes, mood swings, and vaginal dryness.

- Hormone-replacement therapy (HRT) is the treatment currently preferred by most physicians for the treatment of menopausal symptoms.

- There are also natural treatments available that can offer benefits.

Health Risks Associated with Menopause

Osteoporosis and Cardiovascular Disease

A s we saw in chapter 1, the decrease in hormones that occurs during the menopausal years can cause a number of uncomfortable symptoms. The good news about irregular menstruation, hot flashes, and mood swings is that they will pass. However, there are other long-term effects of menopause as well, including some significant health risks. In particular, menopause increases your risk of developing osteoporosis and cardiovascular disease (primarily heart disease and strokes). Fortunately, there is much that you can do to reduce the risk of developing these problems.

Osteoporosis

Osteoporosis is a progressive loss of bone mass and bone strength that often comes with old age. It can cause bones to break more easily and in extreme cases can become a serious physical disability. The word *osteoporosis* literally means "porous bone" (see figure 3), and when the bones

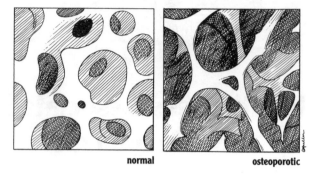

normal   **osteoporotic**

Figure 3. *Normal and osteoporotic bones*

become too porous, they may no longer support the body's weight. The U.S. National Osteoporosis Foundation estimates that 25 million Americans have osteoporosis and that the disease contributes to 1.5 million fractures each year. The majority of these fractures are in the spine (500,000), hip (250,000), and wrist (200,000)[1]—painful, disabling fractures that seriously impair many elders' quality of life.

The word *osteoporosis* literally means *porous bone*. When the bones become too porous, they may no longer support the body's weight.

I worked in a nursing home for many years. Many of the residents in our facility suffered from osteoporosis. I recall one woman who fractured her hip simply by turning her body the wrong way. Many residents were confined to wheelchairs because of their brittle bones.

About 90% of Americans who have osteoporosis are women. However, men are not immune. More than two million American men suffer from osteoporosis. One reason more women suffer from osteoporosis is that although both sexes lose bone mass as they age, men have thicker bones to start with. Men's bones are, on average, approximately 30% larger and more dense than women's.[2] Another reason is that in women the rate of bone loss increases dramatically during menopause, especially during the first few years. Although both men and premenopausal women lose bone mass at approximately 1 to 2% per year, this rate increases to 2 to 5% for postmenopausal women.[3]

While some loss of bone mass is probably inevitable— we don't yet know how to completely prevent it—women today have a number of options for slowing the rate of bone loss and protecting their bones.

Not so long ago, osteoporosis was viewed as an inevitable result of aging for women. However, with advances in medical science in recent decades, we've come a long way toward understanding how osteoporosis develops and how to treat it. While some loss of bone mass is probably inevitable—we don't yet know how to completely prevent it—women today have a number of options for protecting their bones.

The Link Between Osteoporosis and Menopause

Bone is living, vibrant tissue, constantly forming new bone cells and removing old ones in a continuous cycle called *bone remodeling*. Bone remodeling involves two major types of bone cells: *osteoblasts*, which create new bone cells, and *osteoclasts*, which remove old bone cells. The removal of old bone cells and other materials is a process called *resorption*.

The process of bone remodeling—the formation of new bone and removal of old bone—continues throughout our lives. During the first 30 to 35 years of our lives, we make more new bone mass than we lose. Most of us reach our peak bone mass around age 35. After that, the rate of bone removal (resorption) overtakes new bone cell formation, and we begin to lose bone density.

The rate of bone loss at this time is usually between 1 to 2% in most healthy people. This rate can vary; some people are "fast losers" and others "slow losers," for reasons science has not yet identified.

We are still trying to understand all the details of the intricate process of bone remodeling, but there are clear links between menopause and bone loss. For example, we know that several hormones play a role in regulating bone remodeling—including estrogen, progesterone, and calcitonin (produced in the thyroid gland), and all of them decrease after menopause.

Estrogen reduces the rate of bone breakdown. Progesterone, on the other hand, seems to stimulate new bone growth. As estrogen and progesterone decline during menopause, the rate of bone loss increases.

The rate of bone removal is also influenced by the thyroid gland. In addition to producing the thyroid hormone, it also produces calcitonin, a hormone that slows down bone removal. As the amount of calcitonin decreases in our body, the rate of bone loss increases.

Risk Factors Associated with Osteoporosis

Certain women are more likely to develop osteoporosis than others. We know that our genes determine our risk to some degree, because osteoporosis often runs in families. Osteoporosis is also much more common in Caucasian and Asian women than in African American women. The reason is probably because Caucasian and Asian women enter menopause with less bone mass than African American women.[4] Women who are short and thin, who have gone through early or induced menopause, who have high thyroid levels, or who have never been pregnant (nulliparous) are also more likely to develop osteoporosis.[5] We know the reasons why most but not all of these factors lead to a greater incidence of osteoporosis. Women who are short and thin have smaller bones and less bone mass than women who are larger and heavier. The less bone mass you have to begin with, the more susceptible you are to bone loss and osteoporosis. Large-boned people have more bone mass and, therefore, are less affected by increased resorption. Also, fat creates estrogen, so women with less body fat have less estrogen to protect against osteoporosis. Women who have gone through early or induced menopause are more at risk because they lose the protective effects of estrogen and other hormones at an earlier age. High levels of thyroid hormone directly increase bone loss. However, we don't know why nulliparity increases the risk of osteoporosis.

Long-term therapy with prednisone or other drugs in the cortisone family causes severe and rapid osteoporosis as one of their primary side effects. Endurance athletes, or women with anorexia who lose so much weight that their menstrual periods stop, can also develop osteoporosis at an accelerated rate.

Smoking is also believed to increase the risk for osteoporosis. Heavy alcohol use, as well as excessive intake of protein, caffeine, soft drinks, and salt, may also contribute to rapid bone loss.

Positive Lifestyle Steps
On the other side of the coin, good diet and moderate exercise can help prevent osteoporosis. You have to get enough calcium in your diet to build strong bones. It's

Major Known Risk Factors Associated with Osteoporosis

Family history of osteoporosis	Caucasian or Asian race
Small skeletal frame	Nulliparity (never been pregnant)
Hyperthyroidism	Long-term glucocorticosteroid therapy
Anorexia nervosa	Smoking
Low calcium intake	Sedentary lifestyle

never too early to start. Adolescent girls can build for the future by taking in adequate calcium while their bones are still growing. It's important to note, however, that you can't absorb calcium without vitamin D, whether from sunlight, food, or supplements. (See chapter 9 for more information on calcium and vitamin D.)

Exercise also helps to build bone, especially weight-bearing exercises such as walking, running, climbing stairs, and playing tennis.

Reviewing the risk factors for osteoporosis, Ronie said, "Hey, I'm Caucasian, I'm petite, I've never had children, I smoke, I'm a couch potato, and I don't drink milk. Does that mean my bones are going to crumble?" I had to agree that the picture didn't look too good.

Since Ronie can't change her race and size, and it probably isn't a good idea to have children just to prevent osteoporosis, I recommended that she work on the risk factors she could change easily. After researching the issue, she quit smoking and began to take calcium and vitamin D supplements (see chapter 9 for more information on the proper form and dosage of these supplements). She also began to walk two miles a day. Although these lifestyle changes don't guarantee that she won't develop osteoporosis, they will certainly reduce the risk and undoubtedly improve her health in other ways as well.

Specific Treatments to Prevent Osteoporosis

There are many methods of reducing the risk of osteoporosis. Because this is a rapidly evolving and complex field, consult your physician for the latest information.

Hormone-replacement therapy (described in chapter 3) has been shown to help prevent bone loss during menopause. However, it has some risks as well. Newly available "designer" estrogens, such as raloxifene (Evista), work in a more focused manner than ordinary estrogens and may be able to reduce the risk of osteoporosis without creating other problems. There is also some evidence that progesterone may be helpful.

If you wish to use natural treatments, ipriflavone may be your best choice. (Well, *almost* natural: Ipriflavone is a slightly modified version of a substance naturally found in soybeans.) According to numerous scientific trials, ipriflavone can prevent and possibly even reverse osteoporosis. It is described in chapter 8.

Supplementation with calcium and vitamin D is useful, regardless of what other treatments you are using. Other vitamins and minerals may also help. See chapter 9 for more information.

How Do I Know If I Already Have Osteoporosis?

Unlike the more temporary symptoms of menopause—hot flashes, mood swings, and so forth—bone loss is a gradual change that you are unlikely to notice until it has advanced over several years.

Norma, one of the residents at the nursing home where I worked, had been brought to the facility after breaking her hip. Previously, she had always been in good health and was completely shocked to find that she had osteoporosis. Norma did quite well in physical therapy, and after 1 month, she was able to leave the nursing facility and return home. As Norma found, osteoporosis can develop for years without producing any noticeable symptoms.

The hip isn't the only bone that can fracture. Spinal vertebrae can break as well. This can cause severe pain, although it can also be painless, and it can lead to severe curvature of the spine ("dowager's hump") and loss of height.

Several tests are now available for diagnosing osteoporosis in its early stages, before the bone loss becomes severe.

It's better to catch bone loss before fractures occur! Fortunately, there are several good diagnostic techniques that can identify bone loss early. One of the most popular tests is called dual energy x-ray absorptiometry, or DXA scan. This is a low-dose x-ray technique that is noninvasive, and it usually takes only about 15 minutes to complete. Other diagnostic methods include SPA (single photon absorptiometry), DPA (dual photon absorptiometry), CT (computerized tomography) scans and various urine tests. Talk to your physician about which test is best for you. It's very important that you check your bones. In this case, what you don't know can definitely hurt you!

If You Already Have Osteoporosis

If you already have osteoporosis, there are still a number of positive steps you can take. All of the treatments described for preventing osteoporosis are useful in treating it as well. At the very least, they may prevent osteoporosis from getting worse, and they may actually help you grow some new bone. In addition, the drugs Fosamax (alendronate sodium) and calcitonin have been shown to increase bone mass.

Cardiovascular Disease

The other major long-term risk associated with menopause is cardiovascular disease (heart disease, strokes, and
related problems). Cardiovascular disease is the number
one killer of postmenopausal women in the United States.
Approximately 245,000 women died of heart disease in
1996, and another 90,000 women died of stroke.[6]

Menopause dramatically increases a woman's risk for
heart disease and stroke. Prior to menopause, women are
50% less likely than men to suffer from cardiovascular disease. After menopause, however, the risk for women increases until it is nearly equal to that for men.

It appears that estrogen is the primary influence protecting premenopausal women from cardiovascular disease. When estrogen levels drop during menopause, this
protective effect decreases. This is one of the primary reasons given for recommending hormone-replacement therapy (HRT) for women after menopause. However, as we
will discuss in chapter 3, this subject is complex and
rapidly evolving.

There are many other factors involved in cardiovascular disease. In the remainder of this chapter I will summa-
rize them briefly. For more detailed information on
conventional and natural approaches, see *The Natural
Pharmacist Guide to Heart Disease Prevention.*

What Causes Cardiovascular Disease?

Both strokes and heart attacks are primarily caused by the
buildup of plaque in the arteries (hardening of the arteries). The process whereby plaque develops is called *atherosclerosis* (see figure 4).

Atherosclerotic plaque can deprive the heart of sufficient
oxygen, causing the squeezing chest pain called *angina*.
Blood clots may build up on the plaque and then break off,
plugging an artery completely. This causes a heart attack.

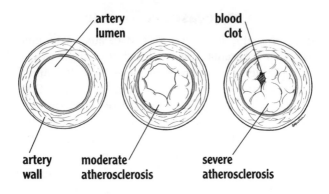

Figure 4. *Cross section of three coronary arteries*

When blood vessels in the brain are completely blocked, a stroke occurs. Temporary blockage or severe narrowing of the vessels without blockage causes a temporary stroke called a TIA (transient ischemic attack), the brain's equivalent of angina.

Medical scientists have not conclusively defined how and why arteries become blocked by plaque. The most popular theory is that atherosclerosis results from an injury to the cells in the lining of the artery. According to this theory, the cells lining the artery are harmed by circulating chemicals such as cholesterol, as well as by the physical stress of hypertension (high blood pressure). This damage causes a complex series of events to ensue, leading to a thickening of the artery wall and a buildup of fat and cholesterol inside it.

Risk Factors for Cardiovascular Disease

Once you enter menopause, you are more at risk for heart disease and stroke than before. But your exact chances depend to a great extent on other factors. The major known

Katie's Story

Katie is an athletic woman who eats a lowfat diet, exercises regularly, doesn't smoke cigarettes, and has good cholesterol levels, low blood pressure, and no family history of heart disease. Overall, her risk of cardiovascular disease is quite small, whether or not she takes estrogen.

Laura, however, was a sobering prospect. Her mother died of a stroke at age 54. When I first met her, Laura ate a diet high in fat, smoked two packs of cigarettes a day, and didn't exercise at all. To make matters worse, because breast cancer ran in her family, her physician did not want to put her on estrogen therapy.

"Without estrogen, and with all these risk factors, you're at real risk," he told her.

"I feel like my life is ending," she said to me, sometime after the appointment. Do I have to give up everything that I like just because there's less estrogen in my blood?" But the more she researched the subject, the more she realized that she had to do something.

Today, Laura takes much better care of herself. She has quit smoking, learned how to cook healthy but tasty food, and started to exercise. She now stands a good chance of living a long, healthy life.

risk factors associated with cardiovascular disease are elevated blood cholesterol, hypertension (high blood pressure), obesity, a sedentary lifestyle, diabetes, and smoking. The more of these factors apply to you, the closer attention you need to pay to the health of your heart and arteries.

Elevated Blood Cholesterol

High levels of cholesterol in the blood dramatically increase the rate of atherosclerosis. There are two major types of cholesterol: low-density lipoproteins (LDL) and high-density lipoproteins (HDL). LDL is often referred to as "bad cholesterol" because it stimulates atherosclerosis. By contrast, HDL's denser molecules do not stimulate atherosclerosis; in fact, for reasons that aren't fully understood, they actually help prevent it. This is why HDL is called "good cholesterol."

Another type of cholesterol that may cause even more damage than LDL is called lipoprotein(a), or Lp(a). It is similar to LDL, but with an additional protein molecule that acts as an adhesive. Several studies have suggested that increased levels of Lp(a) in the blood may significantly increase your risk for heart disease.[7]

Cholesterol levels are usually checked during routine physical exams. I always ask my doctor for a copy of the results, so I can see for myself how high or low my cholesterol levels are. Women with a total blood cholesterol level above 200 milligrams/deciliter (mg/dL) and an LDL level above 130 mg/dL are thought to be at increased risk for developing cardiovascular disease. Ideally, a woman's HDL level should be above 35 mg/dL, and the lipoprotein(a) level should be below 30 mg/dL. The ratio of LDL to HDL should be no higher than 4:1.

Increasing exercise and lowering your intake of foods containing saturated fats will almost certainly reduce your LDL and total cholesterol levels. There are also several natural supplements that can help, such as the herb garlic (see chapters 7 and 10 for more information on these treatments). In severe cases, drug treatment may be necessary to lower cholesterol levels. For more detailed information on cholesterol and how to lower it, see *The Natural Pharmacist Guide to Garlic and Cholesterol.*

Hypertension (High Blood Pressure)

Hypertension or high blood pressure affects more than 60 million Americans, nearly half of whom are women. The American Heart Association notes that half of all post-menopausal women have hypertension. Hypertension damages the arterial wall directly, by physically stressing it, and increases the risk for cardiovascular disease. The Framingham Study, which began in the 1940s and continues today, conclusively showed that blood pressures over 140/90 mm Hg (millimeters of mercury) lead to an increased occurrence of heart disease and stroke. Recent emphasis suggests that blood pressure should be even lower, perhaps 120/80, for optimum heart health.

The best way to control blood pressure is to increase exercise, quit smoking, and lose weight. Cutting back on dietary salt is helpful for some but not all people with hypertension. If you can't control your blood pressure through these natural approaches, medical therapy is recommended.

Obesity

People who have excess body fat are more likely to develop heart disease and stroke even if they have no other risk factors. Losing as little as 10 to 20 pounds will help lower your heart disease risk.

Sedentary Lifestyle

Lack of physical activity is a risk factor for cardiovascular disease. Regular, moderate-to-vigorous exercise plays a significant role in preventing heart and blood vessel disease. Even modest levels of low-intensity physical activity are beneficial if done regularly and long-term. Exercise can help control blood cholesterol, diabetes, and obesity as well as help to lower blood pressure in some people.

Diabetes

Diabetes is a serious risk factor related to heart disease; it doubles a woman's risk of developing heart disease. Nearly 80% of

people with diabetes ultimately die of a heart attack.[8] The best defense is good blood sugar control, along with taking all the other heart-healthy steps that would be helpful for those without diabetes.

An increased intake of fruits and vegetables is strongly associated with a lower risk of heart disease.

Smoking

According to the American Heart Association, smokers have two to four times the risk of nonsmokers of sudden cardiac death.[9] Smoking cigarettes strongly accelerates the development of atherosclerosis, not to mention lung cancer and emphysema. The bottom line: Quit smoking as soon as you can!

Preventing Cardiovascular Disease

The most obvious way of preventing cardiovascular disease is to reduce the risk factors just described. But there are other steps you can take as well. An increased intake of fruits and vegetables is strongly associated with a lower risk of heart disease. The FDA has recently suggested that soy protein can reduce the risk of cardiovascular disease (see chapter 8). The supplement vitamin E may also protect you, and getting enough folic acid and vitamins B_6 and B_{12} will lower blood levels of the harmful substance homocysteine, which is believed to accelerate atherosclerosis. For more information and steps you can take, see *The Natural Pharmacist Guide to Heart Disease Prevention.*

We've seen some of the genetic and lifestyle factors that may increase a woman's risk for developing osteoporosis and cardiovascular disease. But we have yet to consider whether something can be done about the "risk factor" this book is most concerned with: the permanent reduction of hormone levels due to menopause. If menopause increases a woman's risk for these serious long-term health problems, can't she reduce her risk by taking supplemental hormones to increase her levels of estrogen and other critical hormones? As you will learn in chapter 3, hormone-replacement therapy is, in fact, the leading conventional treatment for menopausal symptoms.

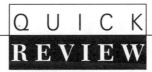

- Menopause increases your risk of developing both osteoporosis and heart disease.
- Osteoporosis is a progressive loss of bone mass and bone strength that often accompanies old age.
- Several tests are now available for diagnosing osteoporosis in its early stages. The most popular is the DXA scan.
- Coronary artery disease (or atherosclerosis) is a result of the narrowing of one or more arteries that supply blood and oxygen to the heart.
- There are many steps you can take to lower your risk of cardiovascular disease: Reduce your blood cholesterol, control your hypertension, lose weight, increase your exercise, stop smoking, and eat a diet high in fruits and vegetables.

Hormone-Replacement Therapy

I f you are entering menopause today, you face a confusing array of data and opinions. For years, conventional medicine suggested as a matter of course that most women start taking supplemental hormones around the time of menopause. Hormone-replacement therapy (HRT) has three goals: to stop uncomfortable physical changes, to prevent osteoporosis, and to reduce the risk of cardiovascular disease. However, there are also safety concerns about this recommendation, and several times a year new studies come out with contradictory information.

To add to the confusion, there are many types of hormone-replacement therapies available, employing different dosages and forms of estrogen and progesterone as well as various other hormones. Even if you are sure that you want HRT, you and your doctor still have to decide which treatment regimen is best.

This chapter will give you detailed information about the various kinds of hormone-replacement therapies available, including their possible side effects as well as their effectiveness. With this information, you will be in a better position to discuss your options with your doctor and to make informed choices about hormone-replacement therapy.

History of Hormone-Replacement Therapy

Hormone-replacement therapy is a term that is used to describe several treatment programs in which a woman takes estrogen, progesterone, or both, or other hormones. Therapy in which a woman takes only estrogen is called *estrogen-replacement therapy* (ERT).

Although scientists first isolated estrogen in laboratories in the 1920s, the use of estrogen to treat menopausal symptoms remained limited for 40 years, until the publication of *Feminine Forever*, a book by New York gynecologist Robert Wilson.[1] Referring to menopause as a "curable disease state," Wilson told American women that estrogen could keep them looking eternally young. The idea struck a chord: *Feminine Forever* became a best-seller in the United States and Europe, and prescriptions for estrogen skyrocketed. The golden age of estrogen-replacement therapy had begun.

If you are entering menopause today, you face a confusing array of data and opinions. To add to the confusion, there are many types of hormone-replacement therapies and many different treatment regimens.

Women were impressed by the power of estrogen to reduce hot flashes and mood swings, improve vaginal dryness, and restore libido. Over time, though, it became clear that ERT had potential drawbacks as well. As early as 1950, the *Physicians' Desk Reference* stated that Premarin (a type of estrogen) should not be given to women with a history of cancer of the breast or genitals. These warnings were dropped after 1955 and not listed again until 1970, when reports of the adverse effects of estrogen therapy began to appear in medical journals and in the news.[2] Studies linked estrogen therapy in postmenopausal women with cancer of the uterine lining (endometrial cancer). Meanwhile, health concerns had emerged connected to the use of estrogen in birth control pills, showing an increased risk of heart disease, blood clots, strokes, and breast cancer.[3] Although hormone-replacement therapy involved much lower levels of estrogen than birth control pills, doctors became reluctant to prescribe HRT for women at risk for cardiovascular disease or cancer.

The use of estrogen to treat menopausal symptoms remained limited for 40 years, until the publication of *Feminine Forever,* a book by New York gynecologist Robert Wilson.

The estrogen boom turned into a bust as the number of women on estrogen therapy dramatically declined. In 1975, 28 million prescriptions were written for Premarin (a common form of estrogen). By 1980, the number had fallen to 14 million. This decline continued until the early 1980s, when research came in showing that estrogen-replacement therapy actually reduced the risk of cardiovascular disease and also appeared to help prevent osteoporosis. Furthermore, it became clear that the combined use of estrogen with a progestin (chemically altered progesterone) significantly decreased the risk of uterine cancer. Doctors began to prescribe combined estrogen/progestin treatment with more confidence. The prescriptions for Premarin rose from 14 million in 1980 to 16.6 million in 1983 and 31.7 million in 1992.

Today there are many forms of HRT available. These include various combinations of estrogen and progesterone and related hormones intended to protect women from cardiovascular disease and osteoporosis while minimizing side effects. Yet there are still many unanswered questions.

Research Findings on HRT and Cardiovascular Disease

Numerous studies have found that women who take estrogen-replacement therapy are almost 50% less likely to develop cardiovascular disease than those who do not. Some of the most impressive results come from the Nurses' Health Study, a long-term observational study involving more than 100,000 women.

In an "observational" study, the researchers don't give the participants treatments or placebos. They just observe, recording such information as diet, exercise, and use of any medications the participant is already taking. The researchers correlate these factors with heart disease and other illnesses. As I will explain further on, there are some significant drawbacks with observational studies. Nonetheless, the results can still tell us a lot.

According to a 1996 report from the Nurses' Health Study, estrogen or estrogen/progestin combinations can reduce the risk of heart disease by about 40%.[4] The combination was about as effective as estrogen alone. The greatest benefits were seen in current users and smokers. Interestingly, the protective effects of hormone treatment start to diminish 3 years after stopping it.

Approximately 25 to 50% of the cardiovascular benefits of estrogen are believed to be due to estrogen's effect on cholesterol levels.[5] Supplemental estrogen is associated with a 10 to 15% increase in HDL ("good" cholesterol), and a comparable decrease in LDL ("bad" cholesterol).[6] There is also evidence that estrogen-replacement therapy may decrease levels of lipoprotein(a), a harmful substance related to LDL.[7]

According to a 1996 report from the Nurses' Health Study, estrogen or estrogen/progestin combinations can reduce the risk of heart disease by about 40%.

However, these changes in cholesterol levels do not seem to account completely for the decrease in deaths from heart disease in these observational studies. Additional protection may result from the direct effects of estrogen on blood vessels,[8] although these are poorly understood.

Keep in mind that there is a significant problem with interpreting the results of observational studies like the Nurses' Health Study. Because researchers did not intervene in participants' lives, hidden factors can confuse the interpretation of the results. For example, suppose that women who take estrogen also happen to smoke less. Then, they will be seen to develop less heart disease, even if estrogen were ineffective in itself!

The researchers who are running this study are perfectly aware of this problem and have endeavored to take the effects of smoking and other factors into account. But there can be hidden factors as well that researchers cannot identify. For this reason, the results of an observational study can never be fully trusted.

To really obtain reliable results, a different form of study is necessary: the double-blind placebo-controlled trial. In such a study, researchers actively intervene in participants' lives, giving them either a treatment or a placebo (a medically inactive substance such as a sugar pill). The purpose of the placebo is to factor out the power of suggestion. For the same reason, the study is "double-blind," meaning that neither doctors nor participants know which group is receiving which treatment.

Unfortunately, there have not yet been many such studies looking at the possible benefits of estrogen in preventing heart disease. One double-blind placebo-controlled study that *has* reported results is the Heart and Estrogen–Progestin Replacement Study, aptly named the HERS study. Its focus is to see whether HRT is helpful for women who already have heart disease.

After 4 years, the preliminary findings of this study have just been released. The results are not promising. Thus far, researchers have concluded that women who already have heart disease should not start HRT.[9] Nonetheless, HRT may still help prevent heart disease in women who have never had it.

Another major study is under way at this time. The National Institutes of Health and the National Heart, Lung, and Blood Institute established the Women's Health Initiative (WHI) in 1991 to study cardiovascular disease, cancer, and osteoporosis in postmenopausal women. The WHI is a 15-year, multimillion-dollar project that will study 167,000 women aged 50 to 79.

This study is very exciting: It will include a double-blind controlled clinical trial as well as an observational trial to examine the effects of HRT, dietary patterns, and calcium and vitamin D supplementation on the prevention of heart disease, osteoporosis, and cancer of the breast and uterus. Unfortunately, the results of the study won't be available until 2008.

Research Findings on HRT and Osteoporosis

Research also suggests that estrogen can prevent osteoporosis. One observational study found that women who took estrogen for longer than 7 years had 50% fewer fractures of the spine than women who didn't take estrogen.[10] The Study of Osteoporotic Fractures examined the risk for fracture in 9,704 women over the age of 65. It was found that women who took estrogen or estrogen plus progestin had 60% fewer wrist fractures and 40% fewer hip fractures than women who had never used estrogen. These are very positive results and strongly suggest that estrogen can meaningfully reduce the risk of osteoporosis.

Testing the effects of HRT on women's health is not a simple task.

However, for women who had previously taken estrogen and stopped, there was no decrease in fractures.[11] These results suggest that taking hormones may protect a woman from osteoporosis, but only as long as she continues to take the hormones.

As we've seen, double-blind placebo-controlled studies are more reliable than observational studies. One such trial examined hormone therapy and osteoporosis: the Postmenopausal Estrogen/Progestin Interventions, or PEPI, trial conducted during the early 1990s.[12] It followed 875 women aged 45 to 64 for 3 years.

The 875 women were each given one of four treatment regimens or placebo. The four hormone therapies tested were estrogen alone, taken daily; estrogen and a progestin, both taken daily; estrogen taken daily only 12 days a month with actual progesterone; and estrogen taken daily only 12 days a month with a progestin.

The majority of women on all four regimens showed an increase of 4 to 5% in bone-mineral density in the spine and a 2% increase in the hip. These women had actually gained bone mass, instead of losing it as adults past their mid-30s generally do.

Putting the results of the PEPI trial together with the results of other studies, we can say with a fair degree of certainty that HRT protects against osteoporosis and can actually reverse it.

Estrogen Therapy: A Closer Look

We have seen that estrogen therapy is believed, and in some cases proven, to be an effective treatment for many symptoms of menopause. In this chapter we've discussed research suggesting that estrogen may help reduce the risks of heart disease and osteoporosis. Estrogen is also believed to be helpful in reducing the mood swings, anxiety, and depression associated with menopause and may help improve short-term memory and reduce the risk of Alzheimer's disease.

Women who took estrogen for longer than 7 years had 50% fewer fractures of the spine than women who didn't take estrogen.

The "estrogen" that women are prescribed today is actually composed of different forms of estradiol and estrone. Estradiol is the predominant estrogen that naturally exists in premenopausal women. Estrone is the predominant estrogen that naturally exists in women's bodies after menopause. A third estrogen, estriol, is considerably weaker than both estradiol and estrone, and is sometimes recommended by alternative practitioners.

Maria's Story

Maria was shocked by the intensity of the hot flashes and mood swings she experienced with menopause. "I never had PMS," she complained, "but here I am angry one minute, crying the next. I feel like I'm on a roller coaster!" Maria tried taking estrogen and found that it worked: Her symptoms decreased dramatically. "I feel like I'm myself again."

Types and Forms of Estrogen

There are many different ways to deliver estrogen to your body. Estrogen is available in oral, transdermal (skin patches), intravaginal (vaginal cream), and injected forms, but the most commonly used form is a simple tablet taken orally. A small percentage of women, however, find that oral estrogen interferes with their ability to digest food or causes other side effects. Women who experience these side effects can usually switch to another form of estrogen therapy.

Oral Estrogen

Premarin, the most commonly prescribed estrogen tablet in the United States is made from the urine of pregnant mares. Most U.S. studies of HRT have used Premarin, so the benefits and side effects of Premarin are better documented than other types of estrogen. Premarin tablets come in various dosages, which makes it easier for a physician to prescribe the right dose for each individual.

Premarin actually contains various forms of estrogen mixed together. Another form of oral estrogen, Estrace, contains only one type of estrogen: estradiol. As just mentioned, estradiol is the most prevalent estrogen in the body. Estrace is not made from the urine of pregnant mares, but rather is produced by chemically modifying substances found in plants. Another estrogen made in the laboratory from plants is esterified estrogen (Estratab), a modified form of estrone.

There are other brands of estrogen besides Premarin, Estrace, and Estratab, but these three are the most commonly prescribed.

Treatment Schedules for Oral Estrogen   In most treatment regimens, estrogen tablets are taken every day continuously for the entire month. Some practitioners prescribe estrogen for only 25 days per month, but there is no proven advantage to the 25-day regimen, and participants often experience symptoms during the days off.

The dose of oral estrogen varies, depending on a woman's general health and symptoms. For preventive purposes, the most commonly prescribed dose of Premarin is 0.625 mg per day. Women who experience severe menopausal symptoms such as daily, multiple hot flashes may require twice this dosage.

Transdermal Estrogen

Transdermal estrogen is taken via a medicated patch applied to the skin. Estraderm is one of the most common brands. This method bypasses the digestive tract, avoiding the digestive distress some women experience with oral forms of estrogen. Another benefit of the patch is that it delivers estrogen continuously instead of in one quick surge, as estrogen tablets do. The patch, which is about the size of a half-dollar, is placed on the buttocks or stomach and replaced every 4 days. Between 5 to 30% of women experience skin irritation with transdermal estrogen, but it is mild in most cases.[13]

Estraderm releases 17-beta-estradiol, which is the type of estrogen the body naturally produces before menopause. Doctors usually prescribe progestins in addition to transdermal estrogen to reduce the risk of cancer (see the following discussion of estrogen's side effects).

Vaginal Estrogen Cream

Vaginal estrogen is primarily used to prevent the walls of the vagina from thinning. However, this therapy does not always restore lubrication: Many women who use vaginal estrogen cream must also use a vaginal lubricant. Like the transdermal patch, vaginal estrogen cream can be used by women who are unable to digest oral estrogen.

Vaginal cream does have its disadvantages, however. The dose of estrogen in the cream is too small to protect a woman against osteoporosis and cardiovascular disease. For this reason, many women who use the cream also use oral or transdermal estrogen. Another disadvantage of vaginal estrogen is aesthetic: The cream tends to be messy and can leak onto your underwear. Most women who use a vaginal estrogen cream use it daily for the first few weeks, after which they apply it only twice a week.

SERMs: The New Designer Estrogens

Selective estrogen receptor modulators (SERMs) are the newest "designer" estrogens. SERMs were created to be the perfect estrogen: a chemical that would produce an "estrogen-like" effect to protect the cardiovascular system and bone density, while having an "antiestrogen" effect on breast and uterine tissue to reduce the risk of breast and uterine cancer.

Twenty-three SERMs are currently being developed, and two are undergoing clinical trials: tamoxifen and raloxifene. Tamoxifen may sound familiar because of the recent news reports that it may protect women against breast cancer. Raloxifene and tamoxifen appear to produce an estrogen-like effect on both bone and cholesterol metabolism.[14]

Tamoxifen is an estrogen antagonist, which means that it blocks the effects of estrogen in tissues, most noticeably in the breasts.[15] Unfortunately, for a variety of complicated reasons, tamoxifen appears to increase the risk of uterine cancer.[16] More clinical studies are needed to evaluate its risks and benefits.

The early research on raloxifene is promising: It seems to have an estrogen-like effect on both bone density while exerting an antiestrogen effect in both the breast and uterus.[17] Its particular value is that it appears to help prevent osteoporosis *without* increasing the risk of breast or uterine cancer. Under the trade name Evista, raloxifene was approved by the FDA in December 1997 for the prevention and treatment of osteoporosis. However, we don't know for sure whether raloxifene protects against heart disease, and it does not relieve symptoms of hot flashes, vaginal dryness, or other physical changes associated with menopause.

Side Effects of Estrogen

Approximately 10% of women who take supplemental estrogen experience side effects. The most frequent are bloating (fluid retention), nausea, breast tenderness, migraines, and headaches.[18] Other side effects include rash, increased growth of facial hair, dizziness, and changes in libido. If you experience side effects from estrogen-replacement therapy, consult your physician. A lower total dose, a different form of estrogen, or a combination with the right amount of progesterone might relieve your symptoms.

Estrone and estradiol both stimulate growth in certain *estrogen-sensitive tissues,* such as the uterus and breast. When they are *unopposed* by the growth-limiting effects of progesterone, estrone and estradiol have both been linked to uterine and breast cancer. This is probably the most serious possible "side effect" of taking estrogen.

Some alternative physicians recommend using estriol instead of other forms of estrogen, in the belief that it does not promote cancer. However, there is no real evidence that estriol is safer than any other form of estrogen when taken in doses high enough to affect symptoms of

Annette's Story

Annette entered menopause suddenly at age 35, when she had a hysterectomy in which both of her ovaries also were removed. Her doctor prescribed hormone-replacement therapy, but she developed severe side effects almost immediately. As Annette said, "I started having hot flashes and nausea. I thought the problems would pass, but then I started having migraines. I couldn't take it, so I just stopped taking the hormones." For Annette, the side effects of HRT were worse than the effects of menopause itself. When her doctor suggested experimenting with various doses of estrogen and progesterone, for a while Annette was too afraid to try them again. Eventually, she did agree and found a combination that worked well for her.

menopause, and estriol does stimulate breast cancer cells in test tube studies.[19]

Progesterone and Progestins: A Closer Look

The terms *progesterone* and *progestins* are often used interchangeably, but they are different chemicals, and their effects can be quite different from each other. *Progesterone* is the actual hormone your body uses to prepare for pregnancy. The term *progestins* refers to drugs that have a progesterone-like effect on the uterus but aren't chemically identical to progesterone. Both types of drugs are manufactured synthetically, but progesterone is sometimes called "natural progesterone" because it is the true hormone your body uses. However, this is a potentially misleading term, since most of us think that "natural" refers to something that is produced by nature, not by a laboratory. In this book I will call the "natural" progesterone you can purchase by prescription or over the counter as "actual progesterone," "true progesterone," or just "progesterone," to distinguish it from progestins.

Progesterone is not easily absorbed orally. Until recently, it had to be used in a skin cream. For this reason, pharmaceutical companies in the 1950s switched over to *progestins,* which are chemical cousins of progesterone that the body can easily absorb. However, actual progesterone has recently come back on the market in a special form that can be absorbed well (micronized progesterone). Thanks to this new technique, it is much more feasible now for a woman to take true progesterone orally.

The term *progestins* usually refers to synthetic drugs that have a progesterone-like effect on the uterus. *Progesterone* is a more "natural" pharmaceutical that is also produced synthetically but nonetheless is chemically identical to the progesterone produced by your ovaries.

The Use of Progesterone and Progestins

Progesterone and the progestins function quite similarly in the body. The most frequently prescribed oral progestin is medroxyprogesterone acetate (Provera). Like actual progesterone, Provera and other progestins protect the uterus from uterine cancer.

The most natural way to use progestins is to take them the last 5 to 7 days of the menstrual cycle while at the same time stopping the use of estrogen. This imitates the natural release of hormones to some extent. However, when you use this method, you will most likely continue to have a period just as you did before menopause, something you may not appreciate.[20]

> **True progesterone does not appear to cause as many side effects as progestins. It may also produce better effects on HDL ("good") cholesterol.**

Another approach is to take a low dose of progestins throughout the month. This does not cause menstruation flow and does seems to protect against uterine cancer, but it can cause unpredictable bleeding or spotting.

Progesterone and progestins are also prescribed for premenopausal women who have midcycle bleeding and are not ovulating, and for perimenopausal women who have excessive uterine bleeding. They may also be helpful for hot flashes and even for preventing or reversing osteoporosis,[21] although more studies need to be performed.

Possible side effects of progestins include depression, fatigue, abdominal bloating, fluid retention, and breast tenderness.[22] True progesterone does not appear to cause as many side effects as progestins, especially the abdominal bloating and fluid retention. Also, in the PEPI trial it produced more favorable effects on HDL, the "good" cholesterol, than standard progestins did. However, true progesterone is much more expensive.

Progesterone Skin Cream

The cream form of real progesterone has been advocated by alternative practitioners as a "natural" progesterone. It

Alice's Story

Alice decided to try HRT for her hot flashes, which were terrible. Her doctor prescribed a typical regimen of estrogen and progestin. But soon after she began the treatment, Alice began to suffer from annoying side effects such as abdominal bloating and swelling of her fingers. She wanted to continue with HRT, so her doctor prescribed true progesterone instead of progestin. Her bloating and fluid retention went away.

is often sold combined with wild yam. However, this is just a marketing gimmick. Although progesterone can be chemically synthesized from substances found in wild yam, wild yam itself contains no active hormones at all.

To make matters worse, many wild yam products claiming to have "natural progesterone" in fact contain *no progesterone at all!* Other products list "natural progesterone" on the label but fail to indicate that their "natural" ingredient was made in a laboratory!

Aeron Lifecycles Laboratory, one of the foremost laboratories in the United States involved in hormone testing, conducted a survey of 27 "progesterone" creams. They found that 11 products had more than 400 mg of progesterone per ounce of cream; 5 products had between 2 and 15 mg of progesterone per ounce of cream; and 11 products contained *less than 2 mg or no* progesterone per ounce of cream.[23]

Not long ago, if you wanted a wild yam–based progesterone cream containing more than 400 mg of progesterone per ounce of cream, you would have to go to a health-care practitioner. Today, on the Internet, you can find creams that contain from 480 to 750 mg of progesterone per ounce of cream, and similar products are appearing in retail stores as well.

The doses of progesterone cream vary from manufacturer to manufacturer. The suggested use of the more potent products (400 mg per ounce) is usually ¼ teaspoon applied to the stomach or buttocks, twice a day.

The effectiveness of progesterone creams is still largely untested. One small study conducted by Dr. John Lee, who strongly advocates the use of "natural" progesterone, suggested that it might increase bone density.[24] However, this study had many flaws and really doesn't prove anything at all. For example, while the participants took a very small dose of progesterone, they also made numerous positive lifestyle changes that may have been more important than the progesterone cream itself.

Progesterone cream can be used for all the same purposes as progestins and oral micronized progesterone. However, it is more difficult to be sure you are getting the exact dose that you want.

The costs of the cream varies: A supply for 1 to 2 months can range from $20 to $32. If you decide to purchase a wild yam or "natural" progesterone cream, carefully read the label to make sure that it contains micronized progesterone, because otherwise it will have no progesterone in it at all.

Major Risks Associated with HRT

We've already seen that some women experience unpleasant side effects from hormone-replacement therapy, especially with the synthetic progestins. But there are more serious potential health risks to consider. Doctors became reluctant to prescribe HRT for certain high-risk women after reports in the 1970s indicated that taking estrogen might make a woman more likely to develop breast or uterine cancer. Medical scientists have been working since then to reduce this risk, first by incorporating progesterone into HRT and more recently by developing new "designer drugs" without estrogen's potential cancer-promoting effects. Yet much remains to be understood about the risks, actual or potential, involved in HRT. We will briefly discuss the major risk factors that are currently recognized.

Breast Cancer

Breast cancer is the most common cancer in women. A 50-year-old woman has about a 10% chance of developing breast cancer during her remaining lifetime.[25] Scientists don't fully understand what causes breast cancer, but one strongly suspected factor is high estrogen levels.

Several studies show an increased risk of breast cancer for women who take supplemental estrogen for a long time—8 to 20 years.[26,27] These studies suggest that taking estrogen over

Studies suggest that taking estrogen over the long term could increase your risk of breast cancer by as much as 30 to 70%, depending on your age.

the long term could increase your risk of breast cancer by as much as 30 to 70%, depending on your age.

However, none of these studies included a randomly selected control group, so it's not certain that the supplemental estrogen was truly responsible for the increased risk of breast cancer. There might have been some unintentional bias tainting the results. Further research is needed to more fully understand this complex issue. The Women's Health Initiative study mentioned earlier in this chapter should give us better information, but those results won't be available for 10 years. Until then, most doctors and other health practitioners recommend that women with a family history of breast cancer or other suspected risks for breast cancer should carefully weigh the risks and

When Is HRT Not Advised?

HRT is not advised for those with the following medical conditions:

- Breast cancer
- Endometriosis
- Uterine cancer
- Blood clotting (thrombophlebitis)
- Liver and gallbladder disease
- High blood pressure (hypertension)

benefits of HRT. If you have concerns, consult your health practitioner. For more information on reducing the risk of breast cancer in general, see *The Natural Pharmacist Guide to Reducing Cancer Risk*.

Uterine Cancer

Unopposed estrogen (estrogen taken without progesterone or progestins to balance it) increases the risk of cancer of the uterus. In the PEPI trial, women who took estrogen alone had a 27.7% increase in endometrial hyperplasia,[28] a pre-cancerous state in the uterus. The same study revealed that using a progestin with the estrogen reduced the risk of hyperplasia. Most doctors now recommend that women add progestin or micronized progesterone to their hormone regimen to reduce the risk of uterine cancer.

Blood Clotting (Thrombophlebitis)

Thrombophlebitis is an inflammation of a vein in conjunction with a blood clot. When a body develops a tendency to form excessive blood clots, this condition is called *thromboembolic disease*. Three large studies have found that women using HRT experienced a twofold increase in the formation of blood clots and pulmonary emboli (blood clots in the lungs).[29] The risk increased for women who took estrogen alone and for women receiving a combination of estrogen plus a progestin. For women who also used birth control pills, which have much higher doses of estrogen, this risk is even higher. As a result of these findings, many physicians recommend that women with a history of blood clots should not take supplemental hormones after menopause.

Liver and Gallbladder Disease

Women with active liver disease should avoid HRT. This is because the liver breaks down estrogen and clears it from the body, so a liver weakened by disease may not be able to perform this critical function. If estrogen is not broken down and cleared from the body, estrogen in the blood may rise to toxic levels.

Hormone-replacement therapy is also not advised for women with gallbladder disease. This is because an excess of estrogen may cause a diseased gallbladder to develop gallstones. Women at risk for gallbladder disease are those who are overweight, have elevated cholesterol, have a family history of gallbladder disease, or have diabetes.

The Choice: Should I Take HRT?

Rose, 45 years old, is starting to think about menopause. She has read several books on the subject because she wants to know what menopause is like before she actually experiences it. As Rose said, "I feel fine, but my periods are beginning to change. I just want to know what to expect, what other women have experienced." She also wants to learn about ERT and HRT, both the risks and the benefits.

Here are some steps that will help you make your decision:

Step 1: Evaluate your own general health, paying special attention to factors related to menopause.

The first thing to do is to have a complete physical exam, including a pelvic exam, PAP test, and breast exam. Ask your doctor for blood tests to check liver function and cholesterol and triglyceride levels. You might also want to get a bone-density test to help determine your risk of osteoporosis. Review your family history with your doctor to assess your risk of breast and uterine cancer, cardiovascular disease, and osteoporosis.

Step 2: Evaluate the benefits of HRT.

Define the phase of menopause that you are experiencing. Define your goals for receiving HRT. Consider the strength of the evidence that HRT will help your situation.

For example, a woman might assess her phase as follows: "I'm in perimenopause and I'm experiencing intense hot flashes." Her goal would be to decrease her hot flashes. She might then examine the success (or failure) of HRT in the treatment of hot flashes. She should also think about long-term issues in light of her risk of osteoporosis and cardiovascular disease.

Step 3: Evaluate your risk factors.

Look at your medical history and the results from your lab tests to decide if you have any risk factors or disease that might mean you shouldn't use HRT. Do you have abnormal vaginal bleeding? Do you have a history of breast or uterine cancer? Do you have an active liver or gallbladder disease? Discuss your possible risk factors with your health-care provider.

Step 4: Compare the benefits of HRT to the risks.

Carefully balance the benefits of HRT and weigh them against the potential risks that you and your health-care provider have identified. Work closely with your health-care practitioner. You don't have to make the decision alone! If you don't feel comfortable making a decision right away, go home and sleep on it. Make sure you feel comfortable about your decision; after all, it's your body.

Step 5: Learn about the full range of available treatments.
Consider other treatments besides standard HRT, including the new designer estrogens and the natural treatments described in this book.

Step 6: Reevaluate your decision as you go.
If you choose hormone-replacement therapy, you and your doctor should periodically review your treatment dosages and schedule to correct any side effects and ensure that your needs are still being met as your body changes. If you develop side effects, notify your doctor. **Warning:** Never stop HRT abruptly, without consulting your doctor! If you choose to stop HRT, your doctor will help you to slowly decrease the medication until it's safe to stop taking it.

Whether or not you choose HRT, chapters 4 though 11 will give you ideas for lifestyle changes and natural alternatives to help you with menopausal symptoms and to generally improve your health.

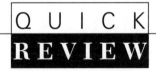

QUICK REVIEW

- Hormone-replacement therapy (HRT) is a term used to describe several treatment regimens in which a woman takes estrogen, progesterone, or both, or other hormones.
- HRT has three goals: to stop uncomfortable physical changes, to prevent osteoporosis, and to reduce the risk of cardiovascular disease.

- Estrogen-replacement therapy (ERT) has been shown to eliminate hot flashes and decrease vaginal dryness. However, estrogen may increase the risk of uterine and breast cancer. Side effects include abdominal bloating, fluid retention, nausea, breast tenderness, migraines, headaches, rash, increased growth of facial hair, dizziness, and changes in libido.

- Progesterone and progestins (chemically altered forms of progesterone) help prevent uterine cancer. They may also reduce hot flashes and prevent and treat osteoporosis; however, more research is needed. Side effects include abdominal bloating, fluid retention, breast tenderness, depression, and fatigue. True progesterone appears to cause fewer side effects than the progestins; however, it is more expensive.

- HRT is not advised for women with the following conditions: breast cancer, endometriosis, uterine cancer, blood clotting (thrombophlebitis), liver and gallbladder disease, and high blood pressure (hypertension). Much still remains to be understood about the risks (actual and potential) involved with HRT.

CHAPTER
FOUR

Herbs

Plants have been used to treat humankind's ills for thousands of years. The World Health Organization estimates that around 80% of the world's population relies on traditional healing methods such as herbal medicine, which uses plants not only for physical healing but to treat emotional and spiritual pains as well.

In our world of modern medicine, we may not realize how much we continue to rely on plants: About 40% of the drugs used today are derived from natural products.[1] Plants have given us hundreds of lifesaving medications such as digoxin, an important heart medication derived from foxglove (*Digitalis* spp.), and quinine, the first cure for malaria, made from cinchona bark. The search continues for new pharmacologically active chemicals from plants. Scientists have studied only an estimated 5 to 6% of all plants for their active substances. So the chances are good that we will discover new treatments from plants.

In the next two chapters we take a look at the most important herbs for treating menopause. You may skip ahead, but first I would like to give you some background information on herbs in general.

Herbs Are Medicines

I have personally seen herbs help hundreds of people over the years. However, I would like to clarify that medicinal plants are, in fact, *medicines.* I've talked to many people who have been led to believe that because a plant is natural, it can't hurt you, and you can safely guess how much to take or for how long. That isn't true at all.

Scientists have studied only an estimated 5 to 6% of all plants for active substances. So the chances are good that we will discover new life-saving compounds from plants.

A woman called me one day with a long list of conditions she wished to treat. I explained that because I wasn't a doctor, I couldn't prescribe herbs for her, and she became very angry. At first, I didn't understand what was frustrating her. I tried to refer her to several alternative practitioners who could prescribe herbs, but she only became more upset. She said, "What on earth are you talking about? Plants aren't drugs, they're natural, so why do you have to *prescribe* anything?" When I asked her to explain just what she meant, she said, "Well, on the radio, a doctor said that herbs are natural, and that you could take as much as you want for as long as you want." She gave me a list of herbs that she had been taking: eight to ten different products on a daily basis!

I spent the next 45 minutes explaining to her what each of them was and gave her information about their long-term implications as well as more general information about what each one actually did. By the end of our conversation, she was shocked: She had no idea what she had been putting into her body.

Medicinal herbs are powerful, and they deserve respect. Yet when used properly, they can be safe, effective medicine.

Herbs and Research

There are numerous herbs on the market today, but only some of them have been scientifically tested and shown to be both effective and safe to use. St. John's wort for depression and ginkgo for Alzheimer's disease are some of the best documented. Several of the herbs I will discuss in this chapter have also been studied in reasonably good clinical trials, although the evidence that they are beneficial in menopause is not yet definitive. I will also cover herbs that have not been clinically proven but that do have thousands of years of traditional use behind them. While traditional use is not as reliable a form of evidence as properly performed scientific studies, it can still tell us a great deal.

Just because a plant is natural, you should keep in mind: Medicinal plants are, in fact, *medicines* and should be treated with respect.

In many parts of the world, herbs are an acceptable part of a health professional's practice. In Germany, physicians prescribe herbs as well as conventional pharmaceuticals. Because of this, some of the best research on herbal medications comes from Germany.

In the United States, research on herbal medicine lags behind pharmaceutical research, partly because herbs are natural products that can't easily be patented. Clinical studies are expensive, and many manufacturers are reluctant to invest their money when they can't get exclusive rights to sell the product. In Europe, however, herb manufacturers have more often chosen to invest money in studies. One reason they have been able to do this is that a proven herbal product can be authorized for use as medical treatment in Germany and other European nations, allowing the manufacturer to recoup its investment. By contrast, U.S. law prohibits the sale of herbs as remedies for specific medical conditions unless they have been approved by the Food and Drug Administration (FDA) as drugs.

In the United States, research on herbal medicine lags behind pharmaceutical research partly because herbs are natural products that can't be easily patented.

Nonetheless, herbal research (mostly using European products) has recently increased in the United States. Today there many U.S. organizations that can provide herbal education and research information to consumers, practitioners, and lawmakers. Organizations such as the Herb Research Foundation in Boulder, Colorado; the American Botanical Council in Austin, Texas; and the American Herbal Pharmacopoeia in Santa Cruz, California are nonprofit organizations dedicated to providing accurate information on the use of botanical medicine. (Information on how to contact each of these organizations is listed in the appendix.)

Herbal Preparations

Walking into a health-food store or pharmacy and looking at the many different available forms of an herb can be a confusing experience. Herbs are sold as crude herb tablets and capsules, standardized extracts, and non-standardized liquid products extracts. How do you know which form to take?

Since most practitioners prescribe tablets or capsules containing "crude" herbs, standardized extracts, or liquid extracts, I will discuss these various forms to help you to understand what you're buying.

Crude Herb Tablets and Capsules

Crude herb tablets and capsules are called "crude" because they are unrefined, raw products. They contain the whole herb or herb part such as the root or leaves, dried, powdered, and pressed into a tablet or placed into a capsule. Tablets and capsules release their herbal compounds via the digestive system, which breaks down the herb and absorbs the chemicals in it. Because your stomach has to digest the herb to draw out the useful chemicals, crude herbs usually act more slowly than liquid herbal products or standardized extract capsules. If you have a weak digestive system, crude herbal tablets or capsules may not give you the full benefit of the herb. The advantage of tablets and capsules, however, is that they're easy to take and easy to carry. Unlike liquid herbal products, tablets and capsules have no taste. This can be a plus factor, because many people dislike the taste of liquid herbal products.

One problem with using crude herbs is that their potency can vary widely from batch to batch. This is because herbs are living organisms composed of thousands of chemicals mixed together, and the exact proportion of each of these chemicals can change, depending on their growing conditions or their methods of storage and processing. Long ago, traditional herbalists got around this problem by smelling and tasting herbs to determine their freshness and strength, and in many cases this craftsmanlike method is effective. But in the modern world, we frequently demand a more objective method of ensuring product potency. Some companies offer freeze-dried herbs, which are fresh herbs that are freeze-dried and then encapsulated. The benefit of using these products is that you don't lose any plant principles that would be lost in the drying process. However, another answer to the problem of varying potency has been developed: the standardized herbal extract.

Standardized Herbal Extracts

Standardized herbal extracts are herbs that have been specially processed with solvents such as alcohol and glycerin (a solvent, usually made from vegetable oils), and then "boiled down" to achieve a fixed percentage of certain ingredients. For example, St. John's wort is standardized to contain a certain amount of a chemical called *hypericin*. While hypericin is probably not the active ingredient in St. John's wort, it is presumed to act as a tag for other as-yet-unknown ingredients that come along with it. More recent formulations of St. John's wort are standardized to contain a fixed level of hyperforin, a substance that may be one of the major active ingredients in the herb.

Keep in mind that standardized products are still different from drugs in that they contain many of the constituents found in the original herb, although in a different proportion than in the raw plant material. Drugs are purified down to a single ingredient.

The big advantage of standardization is that it gives the practitioner and the consumer confidence that one batch of herbs is just as strong as another. However, standardization isn't foolproof. There are many possible methods of extraction, and each can produce a different result. For example, because chemicals dissolve to a varying degree depending on the solvent they are placed in, if one manufacturer extracts St. John's wort using glycerin and another uses alcohol, the percentage of ingredients in the final solution may be very different. Even if the extraction is carried out under different temperatures or for a longer or shorter period of time, the characteristics of the final product can vary enormously. To get around this problem, American manufacturers of standardized herbal extracts have tended to copy the same extraction methods used in Europe.

Some people object to standardized products (especially those from Europe) because toxic solvents such as hexane and acetone are sometimes used in the extraction. However, when prepared properly, all of the solvent is removed during the evaporation process and should not present a health risk. Other people say that a standardized herbal extract isn't really a natural treatment anymore, because it has been processed. But standardized herbs are the products whose claims tend to be backed up by clinical trials, and many practitioners prefer them for that reason.

Unstandardized Herbal Extracts

While standardized herbal extracts are relatively new, for many years herbalists have used unstandardized herbal extracts in liquid form. (Standardized extracts in liquid form are also available.) Generally, water and alcohol or water and glycerin are used as solvents to draw out the plant's active properties. The liquid is not boiled off to achieve a certain percentage of specific ingredients; this type of extract is simply sold with the liquid intact.

One major benefit of liquid extracts over capsules of crude herb is that the body may be able to absorb them better. Another often overlooked advantage is that with a liquid you can fine-tune your dosage more easily than you can with a tablet or capsule. Some people are quite sensitive to very low doses of herbs and medications, so the ability to minutely adjust dosage can be very important.

For example, Mary, who had been diagnosed with depression, is unable to take standard antidepressant medications because she experiences severe side effects. She has a very sensitive body that tends to react dramatically to many substances. Her doctor suggested she try St. John's wort instead, a widely used herbal treatment for depression. Mary knew, based on past experience, that the usual dosage would probably be too much for her so she broke the capsule in half. Yet even this was too much—Mary developed side effects such as anxiety and insomnia. Then someone suggested she try a liquid extract, which she took at a very low dosage—with positive results. "My doctor says that it shouldn't be working at this dosage," said Mary, "but if I take more than five drops a day, I start to have side effects. I know it's not supposed to work, but it works for me, and I'm very happy."

The biggest drawback of liquid extracts is the taste. I've heard some very colorful descriptions of the taste of liquid herbal products. In fact, most people can't stomach the taste and prefer to use tablets and capsules instead.

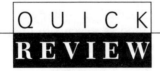

QUICK REVIEW

- Herbs are medicines that have to be used properly.
- Much of the scientific evidence for the use of herbs comes from Europe.

- Herbs come in many forms: tablets or capsules that contain "crude" herbs, standardized extracts, and unstandardized liquid extracts.
- The unique value of standardized herbal extracts is that it is easier to ensure that one batch is as potent as another.
- Liquid herbal extracts may not be standardized, but they offer an advantage in that you can easily adjust the dose.

Black Cohosh

The Best Documented Herb for Menopause

The most scientifically documented herb for treating menopausal symptoms is black cohosh. Studies suggest that it rapidly relieves symptoms of menopause, such hot flashes, insomnia, and vaginal thinning, and produces other estrogen-like effects in the body as well. However, we don't know whether it can help prevent osteoporosis and cardiovascular disease.

What Was Black Cohosh Used for Historically?

Black cohosh *(Cimicifuga racemosa)* is a tall, perennial herb native to North America, originally found in the northeastern United States (see figure 5). Native Americans used it primarily to treat women's health problems, such as menstrual cramps, but also as a treatment for arthritis, fatigue, and snakebite (hence the common name "black snakeroot").

Native Americans later introduced the herb to European colonists, who rapidly adopted it for similar uses. In

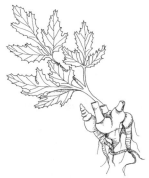

Figure 5. *Black cohosh*

the late nineteenth century, black cohosh was the principle ingredient in the wildly popular Lydia E. Pinkham's Vegetable Compound for menstrual cramps. Migrating across the Atlantic in 1732, black cohosh became a popular European treatment for women's problems, arthritis, and high blood pressure.

Eclectic physicians (doctors who used botanical medications to treat diseases) used black cohosh quite extensively during the late 1800s and early 1900s. In *Specific Medication*, Dr. John M. Scudder wrote that he had excellent results with black cohosh in the treatment of rheumatism. These physicians also used the herb to treat various "menstrual disturbances." The famous Lloyd Brothers

A standardized extract of black cohosh is one of the most commonly used treatments for menopausal symptoms in Germany and other European countries.

pharmaceutical company of Cincinnati, Ohio, at one time manufactured black cohosh liquid medications. It also produced numerous written accounts of the use of black cohosh.

What Is Black Cohosh Used for Today?

Black cohosh is widely used in Germany as an herbal treatment for menopause. In 1994, more than 6.5 million prescriptions were filled. The Commission E (the German government's commission that regulates herbal medicine) recommends black cohosh for the treatment of menopause-related symptoms as well as for premenstrual discomfort and dysmenorrhea (painful menstruation).

What Are the Benefits of Taking Black Cohosh?

Black cohosh appears to have estrogen-like effects in the body. Clinical studies have found that it can significantly relieve many of the symptoms of menopause, including hot flashes, vaginal dryness, anxiety, and depression. Yet even though black cohosh makes you feel better, it may not produce all the benefits of estrogen. We don't know whether or not the herb reduces the risk of osteoporosis and heart disease. This is frustrating, but there are other alternative treatments that can improve your cardiovascular health and your bone density. Many such treatments are described in chapters 8 through 10 of this book.

In 1994, more than 6.5 million prescriptions for black cohosh were filled in Germany.

Nancy's Story

Nancy began to develop hot flashes and anxiety when she was 45 years old. She was afraid to try HRT because there was a history of breast cancer in her family. A friend suggested that she try black cohosh. As Nancy told me later, "I was willing to try anything! I was having really intense hot flashes, but they were nothing compared to my anxiety and mood swings. I have two children aged 8 and 6, and I could hardly deal with them." Nancy began to take black cohosh. "I didn't feel anything at all," she reported later, "until about 3 weeks after I had started to take it. Then I thought I felt slightly better, but it wasn't much.

"My friend told me to give it more time. I'm glad I did. After about 6 weeks, I felt much better. I was only having an occasional hot flash, but, more important, my mood was much, much better. I found that I was back to my old self and had plenty of patience for my children."

Nancy's experience is backed up by clinical studies that have found black cohosh effective for menopausal symptoms. Keep in mind, though, that we don't know for sure whether black cohosh is safe for women at higher risk of breast cancer.

What Is the Scientific Evidence for Black Cohosh?

Clinical research into black cohosh has been conducted mostly with a standardized extract manufactured in Germany. Research suggests that black cohosh has effects that are similar but not identical to those of estrogen. Not only does it relieve most menopausal symptoms, but according to most studies, it also increases the thickness of vaginal tissues. However, the research record is not as strong as it should be. Although there have been many open

studies of black cohosh (see the following discussion), only one double-blind placebo-controlled study has been published. Furthermore, one recent study conflicts with the results of previous research.

> **In a study of 629 menopausal women, black cohosh brought about significant improvement in 80% and complete relief in 50% of the participants.**

Open Studies

A study of 629 menopausal women evaluated the effectiveness of standardized black cohosh in the treatment of symptoms related to menopause.[1] Four weeks after treatment began, approximately 80% of the participants showed significant improvement, while 50% experienced complete relief from their symptoms, which included hot flashes, headaches, nervousness, insomnia, and depression. These gains endured for the full 6 to 8 weeks of the study. The only side effects noted were mild digestive symptoms in 7% of the participants.

However, there was a significant flaw in this study: It lacked a placebo group. It has been demonstrated many times that if a person believes she is taking a treatment, her symptoms are very likely to be reduced, even if the treatment is phony. The best way to know whether a treatment is really effective on its own merits is to use two groups and give one of them (the placebo control group) a placebo instead of the real treatment.

In order to eliminate the power of suggestion, participants and doctors must all be kept in the dark about which treatment is real and which is fake. This is called a double-blind placebo-controlled study. If the participants and doctors are not kept in the dark, the study is called an "open" study. If there is a significant difference between the two groups' outcomes in a double-blind study, then it's fairly safe to assume that the treatment is effective. Open studies are much less reliable than double-blind studies.

Because the study just described was an open study and because it also lacked a placebo-control group, the results are not conclusive about the effectiveness of black cohosh.

Nevertheless, open studies can occasionally provide meaningful evidence. One such study followed 60 participants who were given either black cohosh, estrogen, or Valium.[2] Though all three groups reported a similar level of relief from their symptoms, it's impossible to know how much the power of suggestion influenced these results. However, another change was recorded that can't easily be explained away by the power of suggestion: Microscopic examination of vaginal cells showed positive changes in the women who had received either black cohosh or estrogen, but not in those who received Valium.

Can the placebo effect specifically alter vaginal cells? The answer is that it probably can (see further on). But if so, why didn't it happen in the Valium group as well? The placebo effect shouldn't be able to pick and choose this way! The most likely explanation, therefore, is that black cohosh has an effect on vaginal cells that is similar to estrogen's.

Further evidence for this theory was provided by an open study of 110 menopausal women who were given either black cohosh or placebo.[3] The researchers examined the changes in their FSH (follicle-stimulating hormone) and LH (luteinizing hormone) levels. You'll recall from chapter 1 that both FSH and LH levels rise in menopausal women. In this study, treatment with black cohosh significantly lowered LH levels, suggesting an estrogen-like effect. In the placebo group, LH levels did not decrease.

An interesting feature of this study was that FSH levels remained unchanged. Since estrogen itself reduces levels of both FSH and LH, this finding suggests that black cohosh functions somewhat like estrogen but not identically. Similar results were seen in an animal study.[4] In chapter 8 I will discuss other substances that also resemble estrogen.

> **The best evidence backing up the effectiveness of black cohosh comes from a double-blind placebo-controlled study involving 80 women, which compared the benefits of black cohosh, estrogen, and a placebo for a period of 12 weeks.**

Double-Blind Studies

The best evidence backing up the effectiveness of black cohosh comes from a double-blind placebo-controlled study involving 80 women, which compared the benefits of black cohosh, conjugated estrogen (0.625 mg), and a placebo for a period of 12 weeks.[5] The results were impressive. Not only did black cohosh reduce symptoms so well that the participants said they needed no further treatment, the reported benefits were actually better than those due to estrogen.

In order to measure the extent of the women's improvement, researchers used the Kupperman Menopausal Index, a rating scale that assigns a number to the severity of each woman's symptoms (see table 2).

Table 2. Kupperman Menopausal Index

Hot flashes	4
Profuse perspiration	2
Sleep disturbances	2
Nervousness/irritability	2
Depressive moods	1
Feeling of vertigo	1
Loss of concentration	1
Joint pain	1
Headache	1
Heart palpitations	1

Multiply each number by:

3 if the symptom is severe, 2 if moderate, 1 if mild, and 0 if not present.

Add up the numbers. If your score is greater than 35, you have severe menopausal symptoms. A score of 20 to 35 indicates a moderate level of symptoms, and 15 to 20 means mild symptoms.

Participants began the study with a level of symptoms that rated an average of 30 to 35, or a high moderate level on the Kupperman Menopausal Index. After 12 weeks, participants taking black cohosh reported that their symptoms had declined down to an average level of just under 15, or below a rating of slight menopausal symptoms. In contrast, estrogen and placebo only reduced symptoms down to about a rating of 22, still in the moderate range (see figure 6).

The researchers also looked at the vaginal lining of participants in the study. Surprisingly, placebo treatments produced as much change in vaginal cells as estrogen. However, black cohosh was even more beneficial, significantly enhancing the growth and development of those cells.

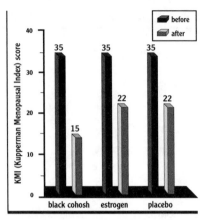

Figure 6. *Effects of black cohosh, estrogen, and placebo on menopause symptoms after 12 weeks in a double-blind study* (Stoll, 1987) *(The lower the score, the less severe the symptoms)*

Finally, the researchers also looked at the effects of treatment on symptoms of anxiety. Again, black cohosh was the most effective treatment, decreasing symptoms by about 50%, a better result than that produced by placebo or estrogen. (See chapter 6 for more information about how we measure anxiety levels.)

One feature of this study is confusing, though. It is hard to believe that estrogen was not more effective than placebo, since it has been found beneficial in numerous other studies. I don't have a ready explanation for this finding.

However, a recent double-blind study reported in the literature of a major manufacturer of black cohosh has confused the issue.[6] This study enrolled 152 women with at least a moderate degree of menopausal symptoms, according to the Kupperman Menopausal Index. One group was given 2 tablets 2 times daily of standardized black cohosh extract, while the other received only half this dose.

In both groups, menopausal symptoms improved significantly and by about the same amount.

So far, the results are not surprising and only indicate that it is possible to get away with a lower dose of black cohosh than was previously recommended. However, the surprise came when the researchers looked for estrogen-like effects in vaginal cells and hormone levels. No such changes were noted. Black cohosh might as well have been water for all the impact it made.

Black cohosh produced changes in vaginal cells and reduced levels of LH in other studies. Why not here? The manufacturers were so impressed by the negative results that they have stopped claiming black cohosh produces effects similar to estrogen. Nevertheless, the conflicting results of a single study does not erase all the previous evidence. Is it possible that the batch of black cohosh used in this study was significantly different from the herb tested in previous studies? This seems unlikely because the same standardized extract was used in all of them, but perhaps there are unidentified ingredients that can vary. Or was there something different about the study design, or the women chosen to participate? Only further research will settle the question.

Dosage

Black cohosh extract is standardized to a chemical called 27-deoxyaceteine. The usual dose is 1 to 2 tablets, taken twice a day, to provide a total of 2 to 4 mg of 27-deoxyaceteine a day. The imported European form of black cohosh is readily available in the United States, and recently, several U.S. companies have also begun to offer black cohosh products; you can find it in both liquid and encapsulated forms, standardized to 27-deoxyaceteine. Unstandardized forms of black cohosh may be effective as well.

Safety Issues

Black cohosh appears to be a very safe herb.

It seldom causes any noticeable side effects other than occasional mild symptoms such as gastrointestinal complaints, headaches, and dizziness.[7] Because such side effects also occur in participants given placebo, they are called "non-specific" symptoms and usually aren't taken too seriously.

Besides side effects, another issue to consider when evaluating the safety of a treatment is its potentially toxic effect when taken in overdose. Black cohosh also seems to be safe in this regard. Studies in rats have found no significant toxicity when black cohosh was given at 90 times the therapeutic dose for a period of 6 months, a time period that corresponds to decades of human years.[8]

Black cohosh appears to be a very safe herb.

Tests have also found black cohosh to be noncarcinogenic.[9] Yet black cohosh appears to imitate some of the effects of estrogen, so it is natural to wonder whether it's use presents an increased risk of breast cancer. Laboratory studies have provided reassuring results. While estrogen stimulates the growth of breast cancer cells in test tubes, black cohosh does not appear to do so.[10] Nevertheless, large-scale studies with real women are needed to confirm whether black cohosh truly does not increase the incidence of breast cancer, and these have not yet been performed. At present, given the apparent estrogenic effects of black cohosh, women who have had breast cancer are advised not to take it. Safety has not been established in pregnant or nursing women or those with severe liver or kidney disease.

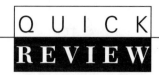

- Black cohosh is the best-documented herb for menopausal symptoms.
- The usual dose is 1 to 2 tablets of a standardized extract taken twice a day, to provide a total of 2 to 4 mg of 27-deoxyaceteine a day.
- Studies suggest that black cohosh reduces symptoms such as hot flashes, anxiety, and sleep disturbances and also normalizes the vaginal wall. However, we don't know whether or not it reduces the risk of osteoporosis and heart disease.
- Black cohosh causes few side effects and is not toxic when given to animals in enormous doses. Even so, it is uncertain whether women who have already had breast cancer should take this herb.

Treating the Anxiety of Menopause with Kava

Many women suffer from anxiety during menopause. This is probably the result of intense fluctuations in their hormone levels, which can make women feel "unbalanced," apprehensive, and nervous. These symptoms can vary from mild to severe. As one woman in the throes of extreme menopausal symptoms said, "It feels like a truck is about to come around the corner and hit me, only I don't know which corner. So I keep looking in all directions. Some days I think my grandchildren are going to get kidnapped, or my daughter is going to lose her job, or I'm about to get breast cancer. I never used to be like this. Sometimes I think I'm going crazy, and my husband is sure I am."

Menopause-related anxiety can be so severe it resembles generalized anxiety disorder, a psychological condition in which causeless anxiety overtakes a person's life. Luckily, the anxiety that is related to menopause eventually goes away, when hormones cease their rapid fluctuations and a woman settles into the post-menopausal period. But if you don't want to wait that long, you might try to find a treatment that can help calm the storm.

Many treatments for menopause in general reduce menopausal anxiety symptoms as well. As I described in the last chapter, black cohosh has been found in one study to reduce these symptoms more effectively than Valium. Hormone-replacement therapy is also frequently very effective (despite the fact that it was not found effective in that same particular study). But there are specific treatments for anxiety as well, and some can be quite helpful.

Menopause-related anxiety can be so severe it resembles generalized anxiety disorder, a psychological condition in which causeless anxiety overtakes a person's life.

The herb kava (see figure 7) is the best documented natural treatment for menopausal anxiety, and it is widely used in Europe for that purpose, as well as to treat anxiety in general. It is a member of the pepper family that has long been cultivated by Pacific Islanders for use as a social and ceremonial drink. The first descriptions of kava came to the West from travelers through the South Seas. They reported that when used properly, kava produced relaxation without intoxication. This interested European scientists, who set to work trying to isolate its active principles. In the 1960s, substances named kavalactones were isolated from kava root and were found to be effective sedatives.

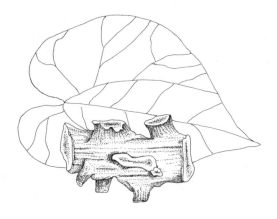

Figure 7. *Kava leaf and root*

What Is Kava Used for Today?

In the words of Germany's Commission E (the German government's commission that regulates herbal medicine), kava can be used to relieve "states of nervous anxiety, tension, and agitation." Although it is not considered powerful enough to treat severe anxiety or panic attacks, kava is often used for milder symptoms of anxiety. For a more general discussion of the uses of kava, see *The Natural Pharmacist Guide to Kava and Anxiety.* The discussion here will focus on using kava to treat anxiety that is related to menopause.

What Is the Scientific Evidence for Kava?

Several double-blind placebo-controlled studies (the most meaningful type of study) have found that kava is effective in the treatment of anxiety. The largest one enrolled 100

Martha's Story

Many menopausal women have told me that they had good results with kava. One woman, whom I shall call Martha, reported that within 1 week her anxiety levels had significantly decreased. "I feel like I can stand my ground again," she says. "Before I took kava, I was as jumpy as a rabbit. Now I have my calm back." According to studies, kava usually begins to work in a few days and reaches its full effectiveness in 4 to 8 weeks.

individuals and followed them for 6 months.[1] Two studies specifically examined the use of kava for menopause-related anxiety.

In the first study, 40 women suffering from menopause-related anxiety received either placebo treatment or 100 mg 3 times a day of a standardized kava extract containing 70% kavalactones.[2] Kava produced dramatically better results than placebo.

In this study, the level of anxiety was measured by the Hamilton Anxiety Scale, or HAM-A. Like the Kupperman Menopausal Index described in chapter 5, the HAM-A assigns a number to match the severity of symptoms. However,

The herb kava is the best documented natural treatment for menopausal anxiety, and it is widely used in Europe for that purpose, as well as to treat anxiety in general.

Table 3. HAM-A Hamilton Anxiety Scale (adapted from the standard rating scale prepared for professionals)

Anxious mood: Worry, hypervigilance, expectation of the worst, turning fears over and over in your mind.

Tension: Feeling tense, keyed up, on edge, easily startled. Nervousness, inner trembling, feeling of restlessness, and inability to relax.

Fear: Unreasonably afraid of being left alone, of darkness, of strangers, of animals, of groups of people, of driving in traffic.

Insomnia: Difficulty falling or staying asleep, not feeling well-rested in the morning.

Impaired thinking: Loss of memory, loss of focus, difficulty paying attention.

Depressive mood: Loss of interest in life, decreased enjoyment of daily activities, early waking, sadness.

Muscular symptoms: Muscle pain, spasm, tension or stiffness, teeth grinding, shaky voice.

Altered sensations: Ringing in the ear, blurred vision, pins and needles, sensation of weakness.

Cardiovascular symptoms: Rapid heart rate, palpitations, irregular heartbeat, feeling faint.

---

it measures symptoms of anxiety instead of overall menopausal symptoms (see table 3).

At the beginning of the study, the participants rated an average of about 30 on the HAM-A scale, indicating a fairly high level of anxiety. After 1 week of treatment, HAM-A scores dropped by 50% in the women receiving kava, and by week 4 their improvement had exceeded 80%. This is a very dramatic improvement and indicates a strong response to treatment. In contrast, only slight improvements were seen in the placebo group.

Table 3. HAM-A Hamilton Anxiety Scale (adapted from the standard rating scale prepared for professionals) *(continued)*

Respiratory symptoms: Pressure or tightness in chest, suffocating feeling, loss of breath, shortness of breath.

Gastrointestinal symptoms: Difficulty swallowing, stomach pain, heartburn, belching, nausea, sensation of bloating, intestinal rumbling, passing gas, diarrhea, constipation.

Urogenital symptoms: Urgency to urinate, frequent urination, loss of libido, inability to achieve orgasm.

Neurological symptoms: Dry mouth, blushing, paleness, tendency to perspire, vertigo, dizziness, gooseflesh, tension headache.

Visible activity (as observed by others): Tendency to fidget, restlessness, pacing, rapid or noisy breathing, hand tremor, frequent swallowing, nervous tics, unusual perspiration, eyebrow furrowing.

Each of the 14 symptoms is rated on a scale of 0 to 4, with 0 representing no symptom and 4 representing a very strong symptom. A rating above 18 indicates a significant level of anxiety.

Interestingly, though we usually think of kava as an antianxiety drug, in this study it also reduced symptoms of depression. From a mathematical point of view, all the results mentioned previously were statistically significant.

The authors of the study suggest that kava should be strongly considered for use in alleviating the anxiety symptoms that often accompany menopause.

Positive results were also seen in another study of the same size performed by the same author, using a different kava preparation.[3]

How Does Kava Work?

Research has shown that kava may produce its sedative effects by affecting a brain chemical known as GABA (gamma-amino-butyric acid).[4]

Research has shown that kava may produce its sedative effects by affecting a brain chemical known as GABA (gamma-amino-butyric acid).

GABA is a naturally occurring brain chemical that appears to reduce anxiety levels. Drugs in the Valium family also affect GABA, though probably in a different way. However, there are other theories about how kava works, and much more research is needed to confirm and better understand its biochemical effects in the human body.

Dosage

Kava products are standardized to contain a fixed percentage of kavalactones.

The daily dose of kava should supply about 140 to 210 mg of kavalactones. Read the label carefully because this might translate into 2 to 6 (or more) capsules a day, depending on how the product is made.

Kava liquid extracts are also available. I like to use them so that I can control the dosage more closely. However, in liquid form, kava has an earthy taste that many people don't care for. It's also a topical anesthetic, so it can temporarily make your mouth feel numb—a good thing to know, because it can be a scary experience if you're not expecting it!

Safety Issues

When used appropriately, kava appears to be safe and causes few side effects. However, long-term use (months to years) of kava in excess of 400 mg kavalactones per day can create a characteristic generalized dry, scaly rash. It disappears promptly when the kava use stops. People with Parkinson's disease are also sometimes warned not to take kava, based on reports (albeit fairly unconvincing ones) that link kava to Parkinson's symptoms.

> **When used appropriately, kava appears to be safe and causes few side effects.**

Kava does not appear to produce mental cloudiness.[5,6,7] Nonetheless, I wouldn't recommend driving after using kava until you discover how strongly it affects you. It makes some people quite drowsy.

European physicians have not reported any problems with kava addiction.[8] However, one animal study suggests that it might be possible to become addicted.[9]

Warning: Kava should definitely not be combined with alcohol, prescription sedatives, or other depressant drugs, as there have been reports of coma caused by such combinations. Its safety for young children, pregnant or nursing women, and those with severe liver or kidney disease has not been established.

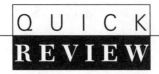

- Anxiety related to menopause is probably the result of rapid fluctuations in hormone levels.
- The herb kava is the best documented natural treatment for menopausal anxiety, and it is widely used in Europe for that purpose.
- The daily dose of kava should supply about 140 to 210 mg of kavalactones. Read the label carefully because this might translate into 2 to 6 (or more) capsules a day, depending on how the product is made.
- Kava should definitely not be combined with alcohol, prescription sedatives, or other depressant drugs, as there have been reports of coma caused by such combinations.
- Kava's safety for young children, pregnant or nursing women, and those with severe liver or kidney disease has not been established.

Other Herbs That May Be Helpful for Menopausal Symptoms

T he herbs described in the previous two chapters, black cohosh and kava, have been specifically studied as treatments for women going through menopause. In this chapter, I turn to herbs that are not specifically aimed at menopause but that may still be beneficial for women going through that time of life. Also, I will briefly mention herbal combination approaches that are widely recommended but that have little or no science behind them.

St. John's Wort: May Be Helpful for Menopausal Depression

Although it is an herb, St. John's wort has recently become the most commonly used treatment for mild to moderate depression in the United States, passing all prescription drugs. It is a low-growing herb that produces bright yellow flowers and is one of the best studied of all medicinal herbs.

What Is the Scientific Evidence for St. John's Wort?

Well-designed double-blind placebo-controlled trials involving a total of about 750 people have found it effective in the treatment of mild to moderate depression, and it is widely used for this purpose in Germany.[1,2] For more detailed information on St. John's wort, see *The Natural Pharmacist Guide to St. John's Wort and Depression.*

Although it is an herb, St. John's wort has recently become the most commonly used treatment for depression in the United States, passing all prescription drugs.

Since depression is a commonly occurring symptom of menopause, women have recently begun to try St. John's wort to see if it will work for them during that period. Although we have no direct evidence that the herb is effective in menopause, it certainly seems reasonable to expect that it might be. Ironically, we do have direct evidence that the antianxiety herb kava can reduce the depressive symptoms associated with menopause (see chapter 6).

I've talked with many women who have used St. John's wort for menopause-related depression. Some of these women used it along with other herbs and supplements, while others used it alone. For example, when Sarah reached 52, her mood took a nose dive. Until then, she had been constantly active but now all she wanted to do was drink tea and stare glumly out of the window. "I was re-evaluating my whole life, and it didn't look like any of it was worth much." Although re-evaluating your life is a worthwhile thing to do, for Sarah it was colored by too much sadness and regret. "It was overwhelming—I was afraid that pretty soon I'd lose my job, and I can't afford to do that."

She started taking St. John's wort and within 6 weeks felt much better. "The lights came back on," she said. Sarah continued to take St. John's wort for a couple of years until she felt she was through the most intense part of menopause. When she stopped, she felt fine. "I think it helped me through the transition," she says.

St. John's wort is generally very safe.

There's no reason to simply endure depression. Whether you use St. John's wort or a prescription treatment, it's important to know that help is available. However, keep in mind that if you become severely depressed, the herb will probably not help you. It is only known to relieve mild to moderate depression.

Dosage

The usual dosage of St. John's wort is 300 mg 3 times daily of an extract standardized to contain 0.3% of hypericin.[3] Some people take 600 mg in the morning and 300 mg at night. Newer products are standardized to 3 to 5% hyperforin instead, but the dose is the same.

Safety Issues

St. John's wort is generally very safe. In numerous clinical studies, the only noticeable side effects reported were occasional allergic rashes, mild digestive distress, and other such nonspecific symptoms.[4]

Excessive doses of St. John's wort can make you get sunburned more easily, especially if you are very fair-skinned. To be on the safe side, if you're taking St. John's wort, you shouldn't subject yourself to artificial UV radiation (tanning beds), and you should take normal precautions against sunburn.

St. John's wort should not be combined with prescription antidepressants. If you have been taking a drug such as Prozac, you will need to let the medication wash out of your system for a period of time before starting the herb.

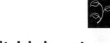

St. John's wort should not be combined with prescription antidepressants.

Consult with your physician about the best way to manage this transition. And if you are taking antidepressants for severe depression, keep in mind that St. John's wort will most likely not be strong enough to replace them.

There are certain other drugs that may possibly interact with St. John's wort. See *The Natural Pharmacist Guide to St. John's Wort and Depression* for more information. Safety for young children, pregnant or nursing women, and those with liver or kidney disease has not been established.

Valerian: An Herbal Treatment for Insomnia

Many women experience insomnia during the transition into menopause. Insomnia can add a great deal of stress to your life, especially if you suffer from it many nights in a row.

Valerian *(Valeriana officinalis)* is a common herbal remedy for insomnia. It is a tall, leafy plant with clusters of fragrant white and pink flowers. Because of its stately beauty, valerian is often cultivated and can be found in many home gardens.

Today, valerian is an approved over-the-counter medication for insomnia in Germany, Belgium, France, Switzerland, and Italy.

What Is the Scientific Evidence for Valerian?

Although the scientific evidence for valerian isn't as strong as it is for St. John's wort, several clinical studies suggest that valerian is safe and effective in the treatment of insomnia. According to the best of these studies, you must take valerian for about 4 weeks before you feel its full effects. In this double-blind placebo-controlled trial, 121 individuals who had a history of sleep disturbances were monitored for 1 month.[5]

Although the scientific evidence for valerian isn't as strong as it is for St. John's wort, several clinical studies suggest that valerian is safe and effective in the treatment of insomnia.

One group was given placebo, while the other received 600 mg of an extract of valerian 2 hours before bedtime. After 4 weeks, the treatment group was sleeping significantly better than the group receiving placebo. However, this effect took time to develop; no real difference between the treatment group and the placebo group was noticed earlier in the study. But once valerian started to work, effectiveness was rated "good" or "very good" by 66% of the participants who received it. In the placebo group, only 29% felt an improvement.

We don't really know how valerian works, but leading theories suggest that GABA (gamma-amino-butyric acid) plays a role.[6] As you may recall from the last chapter, kava and drugs in the Valium family affect GABA, a chemical in the brain that appears to reduce anxiety levels.

Once valerian started to work, effectiveness was rated "good" or "very good" by 66% of the participants who received it.

Dosage

A typical dose of valerian is 2 to 3 g of the powdered herb or 600 mg of an ethanol extract taken 1 to 2 hours before bedtime. The dosage for liquid ethanol extract of valerian is 1 to 2 ml before bedtime. Remember that full effects may take weeks to develop.

I only need to take about 5 drops of extract right before bed to help me fall asleep. If I use more than that, I feel "hungover" in the morning. In fact, you'll know you've taken more valerian than your body needs if you wake up the next morning feeling a little groggy.

Safety Issues

Valerian is listed on the FDA's GRAS (generally regarded as safe) list and is approved for use as a food.

Side effects are uncommon but can include headache, grogginess the next morning, and mild gastrointestinal effects.[7] Strangely, a few people are stimulated by valerian instead of sedated. One woman told me it was like drinking a couple of cups of coffee. The first time you try it, you might want to take a few drops earlier in the day to test its effects on you.

Valerian is a very mild sedative. It doesn't seem to impair your mental alertness or driving ability the morning after you take it.[8,9] However, you may be less alert for the first couple of hours after using valerian so it's not a good idea to take valerian just before you drive or operate hazardous machinery.

Garlic: An Herb That Promotes Cardiovascular Health

As we saw in chapter 2, after menopause you need to pay extra attention to your cardiovascular health, because lower estrogen levels mean you'll receive less of estrogen's heart-protecting qualities. The most important ways to protect your health involve lifestyle choices, such as eating properly and exercising. Beneficial foods, as well as other means for improving your cardiovascular health, will be discussed further in chapters 8, 9, and 10. Good evidence tells us that garlic can also help, by reducing cholesterol levels. It may additionally lower blood pressure and reduce the risk of heart disease in other ways. For more detailed information on garlic, see *The Natural Pharmacist Guide to Garlic and Cholesterol.*

What Is the Scientific Evidence for Garlic?

At least 28 controlled clinical studies that used garlic to treat elevated cholesterol were published between 1985 and 1995. Together, they suggest that garlic can lower cholesterol by about 9 to 12%.[10,11]

One of the best of these studies was conducted in Germany and published in 1990.[12] A total of 261 individuals at 30 medical centers were given either 800 mg of standardized garlic powder daily or placebo. Over the course of 16 weeks, participants in the treated group experienced a 12% drop in total cholesterol.

Good evidence tells us that the herb garlic can reduce cholesterol levels.

Although a couple of studies have shown no benefits from using garlic,[13,14] overall the evidence is strong that standardized garlic powder can reduce cholesterol levels. Garlic oil does not appear to be effective.[15]

Numerous studies have also found that garlic lowers blood pressure slightly, usually in the neighborhood of 5 to 10%.[16,17] Furthermore, garlic may help lessen hardening of the arteries through some unknown influence unrelated to cholesterol or blood pressure.[18]

Many herbs such as vitex, dong quai, licorice, damiana, motherwort, and alfalfa are commonly mixed together into herbal formulas (compounds) said to be helpful for menopausal symptoms.

Dosage

The usual way to take garlic is in the form of garlic powder standardized to contain 1.3% alliin, taken at a dose of 900mg daily. Stated another way, the total daily dose should provide over 10,000 mcg (10mg) of alliin.

Safety Issues

As a commonly used food, garlic is on the FDA's GRAS (generally regarded as safe) list. The only common side effect of standardized garlic powder is unpleasant breath odor. Even "odorless garlic" produces an offensive smell in up to 50% of those who use it.[19] Formal safety studies of standardized garlic powder have not been completed.

Since garlic "thins" the blood, it is not a good idea to take garlic pills prior to or just after surgery or labor and delivery. Also, it should not be combined with prescription blood-thinners such as Coumadin (warfarin), heparin, Trental (pentoxifylline), or perhaps even aspirin. There may conceivably even be risks when garlic is mixed with natural blood thinning agents such as ginkgo and high-dose vitamin E.

Other Herbs for Menopausal Symptoms

Many herbs such as vitex, dong quai, licorice, damiana, motherwort, and alfalfa are commonly mixed together into herbal formulas (compounds) said to be helpful for menopausal symptoms. These formulas are available from many different herb companies, in a variety of forms. However, none of these individual herbs or formulations have been proven effective for menopausal symptoms in proper scientific trials. One of them, dong quai, has actually been shown to be ineffective when used alone.[20] However, in traditional Chinese medicine, dong quai is never used alone. So, it is quite possible that combinations of herbs may produce beneficial effects that are not seen when they are taken individually.

Certainly, many anecdotal reports attest to the effectiveness of these herb combinations for symptoms of menopause. As we have seen, though, the placebo effect can be very powerful. Until proper scientific studies are conducted, it isn't possible to really know whether these traditional herbal combinations really work.

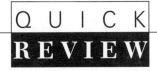

QUICK REVIEW

- St. John's wort is widely used for the treatment of mild to moderate depression. It may also be useful in treating menopause-related depression as well.

- The usual dosage of St. John's wort is 300 mg 3 times daily of an extract standardized to contain 0.3% of hypericin. Some people take 600 mg in the morning and 300 mg at night. Newer products standardized to 3 to 5% hyperforin are taken at the same dosage.

- St. John's wort should not be combined with prescription antidepressants.

- Valerian is a common herbal remedy for insomnia, which may be helpful for menopause-related insomnia.

- A typical dose of valerian is 2 to 3 g of the powdered herb or 600 mg of an ethanol extract taken 1 to 2 hours before bedtime.

- Garlic can lower cholesterol levels and thereby help protect your cardiovascular health. The usual dose is 900 mg a day of garlic powder extract standardized to contain 1.3% alliin.

- Because garlic "thins" the blood, do not take garlic pills prior to or immediately after surgery or labor and delivery. It also should not be combined with prescription blood-thinners such as Coumadin (warfarin), heparin, Trental (pentoxifylline), and perhaps even aspirin.

Phytoestrogens

W e've seen that certain plants, used as medicinal herbs can relieve many of the symptoms of menopause. The difference between herbs and plants that are used as food is somewhat arbitrary. In this chapter we'll look at another class of plant-based treatments for symptoms of menopause. These natural remedies contain *phytoestrogens* (estrogen-like substances from plants). Phytoestrogens are found in a variety of foods, including seeds, legumes, vegetables, and other plant substances. The most common sources of phytoestrogens for medicinal use are soybeans, flaxseeds, and red clover. Black cohosh is also thought to contain phytoestrogens (see chapter 5).

Phytoestrogens may help relieve menopausal symptoms such as hot flashes and mood swings. Some may even offer protection against cardiovascular disease, osteoporosis, and cancer of the breast and uterus.

What Are Phytoestrogens?

Phytoestrogens are naturally occurring plant chemicals that produce estrogen-like effects in the body. They are not chemically the same as the estrogens your body makes, but when digested and absorbed they act somewhat like estrogen in the body. However, this effect is much weaker than your body's natural estrogen.

The most common sources of phytoestrogens for medicinal use are soybeans, flaxseeds, and red clover.

Phytoestrogens actually produce two opposite effects at once. Because this is a confusing idea, I will take a moment to explain it. Estrogen functions in your body by locking on to special estrogen receptors that stick out from cells like tiny phone booths. The phone booth is designed in such a way that only estrogen and chemicals resembling estrogen can enter it. When an estrogen molecule occupies one of these booths (receptors), it sends a signal to the cell that affects how it behaves. In the case of a cell of the uterine wall, the message may say, "Develop and proliferate." To a bone cell it may signal, "Don't break down any more bone."

The problem is that estrogen has both good and bad effects in the body. Not only does it protect bone, it also stimulates the growth of cancer cells in the uterus and breast. This is where phytoestrogens come into the picture. They look enough like estrogen that they can enter the phone booth. Once they attach, the phone booth is occupied, and real estrogen can't get in. Phytoestrogens then send estrogen-like messages to cells, but it is a weaker message. With any luck, the message will be strong enough to produce some of the positive effects of estrogen but too weak to stimulate the growth of cancer cells.

The image I have just portrayed is only approximately accurate. There are other effects at work as well, and much remains to be understood. But the field of phytoestrogens is one of the most exciting and rapidly developing branches of preventive medicine. It offers great promise for reducing osteoporosis, preventing heart disease, and preventing several forms of cancer.

The Three Main Types of Phytoestrogens

There are three main classes of phytoestrogens: isoflavones, lignans, and coumestans.

Soy contains the highest amount of *isoflavones*. Or, it would be more accurate to say, soy contains the highest amount of chemicals that *turn into* isoflavones (see the following sections). As described later, soy isoflavones may reduce menopausal symptoms and also reduce the risk of cancer and heart disease. Similar substances are found in red clover, and a slightly modified soy isoflavone named ipriflavone has recently come on the market as a natural treatment for strengthening bone.

There are three main classes of phytoestrogens: isoflavones, lignans, and coumestans.

Lignans are constituents found in the cell walls of many fruits, grains, and vegetables, and especially in flaxseeds. Lignans may also help reduce menopausal symptoms and reduce the risk of cardiovascular disease and cancer.[1]

The third class of phytoestrogens, *coumestans,* are not thought to be a useful source of phytoestrogens. Coumestans are found in many types of bean sprouts, such as mung beans.

Sources of phytoestrogens are listed in table 4.

In their original form, isoflavones and lignans do not work as phytoestrogens. However, they are transformed into useful substances by complicated changes inside your digestive system.[2] For example, when you eat a flaxseed muffin, bacteria in your intestines work on the raw ingredients and convert them into enterodiol and enterolactone, which have estrogen-like effects in your body. If you take antibiotics that temporarily wipe out these helpful intestinal bacteria, your body will not be able to convert isoflavones and lignans into these estrogen-like chemicals very fast.[3]

Soy is particularly good because it's high in phyto-estrogens and is available in many different forms, which can easily be added to your diet.

Once your body converts the raw material into the estrogen-like chemicals, they can bind to estrogen receptors. As we've already seen, they can actually compete with your body's estrogen by trying to fill the same receptor sites (the tiny phone booths). When estrogen levels are too high, this "competition" appears to reduce the effects of estrogen by replacing your body's stronger estrogen with the weaker phytoestrogen. When estrogen levels are too low, it appears that phytoestrogens simulate the effects of estrogen and partially make up for the deficiency.

Phytoestrogens and Menopause-Related Symptoms

Evidence suggests that phytoestrogens (both isoflavones and lignans) can reduce symptoms such as hot flashes and

Table 4. Food Sources of Phytoestrogens[4]

Isoflavones	Lignans		Coumestans
Legumes	**Whole Grains, Fruits, Seeds, Veggies**		**Bean Sprouts**
soybeans	wheat	apples	alfalfa
lentils	wheat germ	pears	soybean
beans	barley	flaxseed	sprouts
chickpeas	hops	sunflower seeds	
rice	carrots		
oats	garlic		

vaginal dryness. For example, one study of dietary phyto-estrogens evaluated the effects of both soy flour and un-bleached wheat flour.[5] These flours were administered in a random, double-blind fashion to 58 postmenopausal women who were having at least 14 hot flashes per week. Hot flashes decreased significantly for women in the soy group as compared to the wheat group.

When estrogen levels are too low, it appears that phytoestrogens simulate the effects of estrogen and partially make up for the deficiency.

In another clinical trial, 104 women took daily doses of either 60 g of soy protein or placebo. Soy was significantly superior to placebo in reducing hot flashes.[6] Good results were seen by 4 weeks and continued throughout the 3-month trial.

You may not need to take as much as 60 g of soy protein a day to see an improvement in your symptoms. Many women report benefits from 20 g a day, an amount that is easily reached with two servings of soy products. The best thing about phytoestrogens is that you can easily incorporate them into your diet. Nina Shandler's excellent cookbook *Estrogen the Natural Way* has lots of delicious recipes for adding soy and other phytoestrogens to your diet (see appendix).

Phytoestrogens and Cardiovascular Health

In chapter 2, we saw that women face an increased risk for heart disease as their estrogen levels decrease during menopause. Because of their subtle estrogenic effects in the body, phytoestrogens might help make up for this decrease and protect women's cardiovascular health after menopause. Evidence for this theory comes from studies conducted in countries where soy makes up a large part of the daily diet,[7] as well as from evidence that phytoestrogens can lower cholesterol and triglyceride levels.[8]

> Evidence suggests that phytoestrogens (both isoflavones and lignans) can reduce symptoms such as hot flashes and vaginal dryness.

A *meta-analysis* (a combined evaluation of several studies) of 38 controlled clinical trials concluded that eating soy protein can significantly decrease total cholesterol levels, LDL (bad) cholesterol, and triglycerides. The average soy protein intake of participants in the study was 47 grams a day.[9]

A recent study compared the effects of a diet set by the National Cholesterol Education Program (NCEP) to the exact same diet plus soy protein containing 56 mg total isoflavones, and to the same diet plus soy protein containing 90 mg of isoflavones. Although total cholesterol levels did not change, there were significant decreases in LDL ("bad" cholesterol) and significant increases in HDL ("good" cholesterol) in the soy groups.[10]

Further studies are needed to confirm these findings and to understand the mechanisms by which soy and other phytoestrogens work in the body. But these plant-based substances—especially soy— definitely hold great promise for the prevention of heart disease. The evidence is so encouraging that at the time of this writing, the FDA has recommended that foods containing soy protein should carry a "heart-healthy" label.

Soy comes in many forms. Some people enjoy eating soy nuts as a snack or adding soy milk to cereals and beverages. The FDA states that 25 g of soy protein a day are enough to provide some benefit for the heart. This amount is about equal to 2 soy burgers, ½ of a standard block of tofu, or 2½ cups of soy milk daily. Check the labels on soy products to see how much soy protein you get with each serving.

Because of their subtle estrogenic effects in the body, phytoestrogens might help make up for the decrease in estrogen and protect women's cardiovascular health after menopause.

Ipriflavone and Osteoporosis

At the present time, we don't have much evidence that soy can reduce the risk of osteoporosis. However, a chemically modified version of a soy isoflavone named *ipriflavone* has been extensively studied and has become an accepted treatment for osteoporosis in Italy, Turkey, and Japan. It is available in over 22 countries and in most drugstores in the United States as a nonprescription dietary supplement.

Ipriflavone appears to function like estrogen in its ability to slow bone breakdown by inhibiting the growth of osteoclasts, the cells that reabsorb bone. But it does not seem to have estrogenic effects anywhere else in the body. For this reason, it does not reduce hot flashes, night sweats, mood changes, or vaginal dryness and probably does not reduce the risk of heart disease or raise the risk of cancer.

What Is the Scientific Evidence for Ipriflavone?

Numerous double-blind placebo-controlled studies involving a total of over 1,000 participants have examined the effects of ipriflavone on osteoporosis.[11–15] Overall, it appears that ipriflavone can stop the progression of osteoporosis and perhaps reverse it to some extent.

A chemically modified version of a soy isoflavone named _ipriflavone_ has been extensively studied and has become an accepted treatment for osteoporosis in Italy, Turkey, and Japan.

For example, a 2-year double-blind placebo-controlled study of 453 postmenopausal women with bone loss found that ipriflavone was able to reverse bone loss in the spine.[16] The ipriflavone-treated women had a 0.4% gain of spinal bone density, while in the placebo group there was a net loss of 1 to 2%. The difference may sound small but it can add up to a lot of bone over time.

A combination treatment with calcium may be even more beneficial. In one study, 60 women who had already been diagnosed with osteoporosis and had already suffered one spinal fracture were given either 1,000 mg of calcium or 1,000 mg of calcium with ipriflavone.[17] After 6 months, the ipriflavone group had an increase of bone density in the spine of 3.5%. The calcium alone group had a decrease in spinal bone density of 2.1%.

Finally, combining ipriflavone with estrogen may produce even greater benefits in osteoporosis than estrogen alone.[18] However, we do not know whether such combinations enhance or impair estrogen's other benefits, such as reducing heart disease.

Dosage
The proper dose of ipriflavone is 200 mg 3 times daily or 300 mg 2 times daily.

Safety Issues
In clinical studies enrolling thousands of women, ipriflavone has not been associated with any significant side effects. However, individuals with severe kidney disease should take ipriflavone (or any other supplement) only on the advice of a physician. Finally, although ipriflavone is not believed to increase the risk of cancer, women who have already had breast cancer should use ipriflavone only on the advice of a physician.

Phytoestrogens and Cancer
Phytoestrogens may also reduce the risk of cancer of the breast and uterus. These cancers tend to depend on estrogen to grow. By "getting in the way" of more powerful natural estrogens, phytoestrogens may deprive these cancers of their support and stop them from getting started.[19,20] (There are also other theories on how phytoestrogens may prevent cancer.)

Phytoestrogens and Breast Cancer

Soy may reduce the risk of breast cancer. One Chinese study investigated 200 premenopausal women who had breast cancer, and 420 similar women who did not have breast cancer. They each filled out a food questionnaire about what they'd eaten during the year before the interview. Women who ate more animal protein were more likely to have breast cancer than the women who ate more soy protein.[21]

Phytoestrogens may also reduce the risk of cancer of the breast and uterus.

A similar study in the United States looked at 144 pre- and postmenopausal women with newly diagnosed breast cancer and compared them to women without cancer who were similar in other respects. Again, each participant completed a dietary questionnaire. The levels of phytoestrogens in their urine were measured as well. The results of this study suggested that women who ingested high levels of phytoestrogens were at a substantially lower risk for breast cancer.[22]

However, both of these studies are of a type called "retrospective." They look back at what happened in the past. In such studies, it is hard to tell which aspects of a participant's life really made the difference. Studies are more meaningful when they follow people into the future and, even better, involve giving the participants a specific therapy. Presently, several studies of this type are in progress. We should soon know more about whether soy and other phytoestrogens can actually prevent cancer.

We don't know the optimum cancer-fighting dose of phytoestrogens. However, a good suggestion is to eat at least 25 g of soy protein daily.

Phytoestrogen Supplements

Adding plant-based foods to your diet isn't feasible for everyone. Maya, for example, was a businesswoman who spent a lot of time on the road. "I just don't have time to cook," she complained. "Most of the restaurants that I go to on my business trips don't offer tofu. I tried to use flaxseed oil, but that had to stay refrigerated, so I couldn't bring that on my trips." For women like Maya, it's a good thing that phytoestrogens can be taken in the form of tablets or capsules. Several phytoestrogen supplements are currently on the market, and new ones are always being introduced.

What If I Don't Like Eating Soy Foods?

As we've seen, phytoestrogens can be powerful in treating a wide range of health concerns and symptoms related to menopause, from hot flashes to cardiovascular disease and cancer. But not everyone likes eating soy. Ipriflavone is another choice, but it only seems to be effective for osteoporosis. Recently, supplements have come on the market that contain concentrated phytoestrogens, primarily isoflavones.

One of the newer arrivals is an extract of red clover blossoms (*Trifolium pratense*) standardized to contain 40 mg of isoflavones (genistein, diadzein, formononetin, and biochanin-A) per capsule. This type of product has become the leading dietary supplement for menopause in Australia. According to unpublished studies from Australia, these products are quite effective at reducing menopausal symptoms, and they produce no significant side effects when used as directed. Remember: As with

Chrissy's Story

Chrissy was beginning to experience symptoms associated with menopause. She had heard about soy as an effective treatment for hot flashes and other menopause-related symptoms, so she bought several books on the subject. After spending a month or two reading her books, she decided to add two to three servings of soy to her daily diet. Because Chrissy can't stand tofu, she chose to add soy milk, soy burgers, and other soy products to her diet. After 8 weeks, she was pleased to notice a decrease in the number of hot flashes she experienced.

any medicine (herbal or drug), it's important to not exceed the recommended dosage.

Dr. Lila Nachtigall, a professor of obstetrics and gynecology at the New York School of Medicine, is currently conducting clinical trials of this red clover supplement in the United States. The recommended dosage is 1 tablet a day, which will give you 40 mg of isoflavones. If you choose to take other products that contain isoflavones, this same dosage is probably good to aim for.

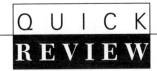

QUICK REVIEW

- Phytoestrogens are naturally occurring plant chemicals that produce estrogen-like effects in the body, which may help reduce menopausal symptoms such as hot flashes, vaginal dryness, anxiety, and mood swings.

- Phytoestrogens may reduce your risk of developing cardiovascular disease, osteoporosis, and certain estrogen-dependent cancers, including breast cancer.

- Although phytoestrogens are found in various fruits and vegetables, soybeans and flaxseeds are the most common sources.

- Adding 25 g of soy protein a day to your diet can reduce your cholesterol levels. This is about equal to 2 soy burgers, ½ of a standard block of tofu, or 2½ cups of soy milk daily. The same dose may reduce hot flashes and might reduce the odds of getting certain cancers, such as breast and uterine cancer.

- Strong scientific evidence suggests that the chemically modified isoflavone named ipriflavone can prevent or even reverse osteoporosis. The proper dose is 200 mg 3 times daily or 300 mg 2 times daily. Taking calcium along with ipriflavone may produce even better results.

- New concentrated isoflavone products have recently come on the market. A typical daily dose supplies 40 mg of isoflavones.

Vitamins, Minerals, and Other Supplements

S o far we've discussed a number of natural therapies that can help relieve some of the uncomfortable symptoms of menopause and also reduce some of the long-term risks such as osteoporosis, cardiovascular disease, and cancer. In this chapter we'll explore the use of vitamins, minerals, and other food supplements in menopause. As we will see, some may help prevent osteoporosis and heart disease, but there is no real evidence that any of them can reduce menopausal symptoms.

Calcium and Vitamin D: Definitely Helpful for Osteoporosis

Calcium is necessary to build and maintain bone. In fact, every cell in your body needs calcium. It helps keep your heart beating, plays a role in maintaining normal blood pressure, and is essential for muscle contraction. It also regulates the transport of ions (electrically charged particles) across cell membranes, making it particularly important in nerve transmission. Furthermore, you are constantly losing calcium through your kidneys. You need to take in enough calcium to make up for your losses and meet all these needs.

Calcium is so essential that your body will never let the level of calcium in your blood fall below a certain point. If you begin to run short on calcium, your skeleton serves as a "calcium bank," which means that your body will "borrow" calcium from your bones as needed. Obviously, if your body repeatedly steals calcium from your bones, your bone mass will diminish. For this reason, no matter what treatment for osteoporosis you use, you need to get enough calcium.

Every cell in your body needs calcium. It helps keep your heart beating, plays a role in maintaining normal blood pressure, and is essential for muscle contraction.

But to absorb calcium, you also need vitamin D. Without vitamin D, calcium will remain in your digestive tract unutilized, and the calcium that is in your body will not be processed normally. Vitamin D is unusual among vitamins, because your body can manufacture it when the sun strikes your exposed skin. (Most vitamins come only from food.) However, if you live in the northern latitudes, spend much of your time indoors, or always wear sunblock, you may not be able to make enough vitamin D this way, and supplements may be necessary.

If you do get enough vitamin D and calcium, you will be less likely to develop osteoporosis. This is true whether you take estrogen or not.

Ann's Story

Ann is 62 years old and already is experiencing signs of osteoporosis. Even though there is no breast cancer in her family, her mother and grandmother both broke their hips in later life due to osteoporosis. Ann was eager to take estrogen. "I have a lot left to do in my life," she says. "I don't have time for any broken hips or getting all stooped over." But she wasn't satisfied just to take estrogen. "I want to do everything that's good for me," she says.

After consulting with her physician, who takes an interest in nutritional matters, she started drinking two glasses of calcium-fortified orange juice daily and taking an additional 500 mg of calcium in pill form, for a total daily intake of 1,000 mg. She figures she gets a little more in the form of cheese and milk (which she doesn't much like), so all together it should be plenty. She also takes a multivitamin and mineral supplement to get the trace minerals she needs. In addition, she takes a separate vitamin D tablet, giving her a total of 800 IU (international units) of vitamin D daily. This is rather high, but her physician has advised it. "I never get out in the sun at all without SPF 50 block on. I've had skin cancer twice. So my doctor thinks I need to take this much."

Is Ann doing everything she should? Perhaps, but there are a few more possibilities. Perhaps the most important is to get enough exercise, as discussed in chapter 10. "I'm a couch potato," she says. "But my doctor is working on that, and I suppose he's right."

What Is the Scientific Evidence for Calcium?

Numerous reliable studies indicate that calcium supplements can help slow or help prevent osteoporosis.[1] When taken at the recommended doses, calcium seems to be able to reduce bone loss in postmenopausal women in every bone site except the spine.[2,3]

When vitamin D is taken along with calcium, the results can be even better.[4] Some studies have found that the combination can reverse osteoporosis to a small extent.[5,6]

Estrogen therapy produces a more powerful effect on osteoporosis than calcium and vitamin D. However, if you take estrogen, you should take calcium (and probably vitamin D) as well.[7,8] The treatments seem to work well together.

The best time to begin the fight against osteoporosis may be in childhood. Evidence suggests that calcium supplements help adolescent girls "put calcium in the bank."[9] The more bone mass you build while you are young, the less likely you are to develop osteoporosis. We reach peak bone mass in our mid-30s, so there is plenty of time to prepare.

Adding various trace minerals (zinc, 15 mg; copper, 2.5 mg; and manganese, 5 mg) along with calcium and vitamin D may produce further improvement.[10,11]

Dosage

Appropriate dietary intake of calcium is as follows: 400 mg daily for infants; 800 mg daily for children up to the age of

> **The best time to begin the fight against osteoporosis may be in childhood. Evidence suggests that calcium supplements help adolescent girls "put calcium in the bank."**

19; 1,000 mg daily for adults up to the age of 50; and 1,200 mg per day for adults over 50 as well as for pregnant or nursing women. Because calcium competes with the absorption of other minerals, you should consider taking a multimineral supplement along with it.

The usual recommendation for vitamin D is 400 IU (international units) daily. However, some of the studies cited here used doses as high as 800 or 1,000 IU daily. Such doses should be taken only with medical supervision.

Sources of Calcium and Vitamin D

Calcium is found in many different foods. Some of the best sources are listed in table 5. As you can see, milk is not the

only option, although it is one of the best. Calcium-fortified soy milk, orange juice, and tofu are also very rich in calcium, as are canned sardines, various legumes, and dark green vegetables.

Oyster shells, dolomite, and bonemeal are inexpensive sources of calcium, but they may contain lead.

Another option is calcium supplements. However, there are so many different forms of calcium supplements available, it can be bewildering. To help you choose among the bewildering array of calcium products, here is a brief description of the major forms of calcium available today and their pros and cons.

Oyster Shell, Dolomite, and Bonemeal

Many people prefer these forms of calcium because they're very inexpensive. However, these supplements have a serious shortcoming: Many of them may contain high levels of lead. The United States Food and Drug Administration (FDA) only allows 1 mcg of lead per 800 mg of calcium, but many products exceed this amount. Some

Table 5. Good Food Sources of Calcium[12]

Source	Serving size	Content in mgs
Dairy		
Milk, whole	1 cup	290 mg
Milk, lowfat, 2%	1 cup	300 mg
Cottage cheese	1 cup	130 mg
Cheese, jack	1 oz.	212 mg
Yogurt, lowfat plain	1 cup	415 mg
Yogurt, whole milk	1 cup	275 mg
Other Beverages		
Calcium-fortified orange juice	1 cup	200–300mg
Calcium-fortified soymilk	1 cup	200–300 mg
Fish		
Sardines, canned (with bones)	3 oz.	372 mg
Salmon, canned (with bones)	4 oz.	90 mg
Oysters	4 oz.	107 mg
Vegetables		
Kale	½ cup	74mg
Broccoli	½ cup	68 mg
Collard greens	½ cup	105 mg
Mustard greens	½ cup	97 mg
Beans		
Black-eyed peas	1 cup	212 mg
Calcium-set tofu	1 cup	310 mg
Hummus	½ cup	62 mg

manufacturers have their products certified by an independent laboratory to verify that their product is safe. If you want to use one of these supplements, check its label to make sure it's been certified to contain a "safe" amount of lead (no more than the FDA's limit).

Calcium Carbonate

Calcium carbonate is a very inexpensive form of calcium, and it's one of the most practical in terms of how many pills you need to take daily to get your daily requirement. However, it can cause constipation, gas, and bloating. Furthermore, calcium carbonate is not absorbed well unless you have adequate amounts of acid in your stomach. Because stomach acid secretion often decreases with age, and many women take drugs such as Zantac to reduce stomach acid, calcium carbonate may not be the best form for you. If you do use this type of calcium, take it with food, because the natural acid secretion that goes along with a meal will improve its absorption considerably.

Calcium Citrate

Calcium citrate may be easier for your body to absorb than calcium carbonate. However, you have to take a lot more of it to get the same amount of calcium. The daily dose may be as much as six large tablets. Also, it's more expensive than calcium carbonate.

Calcium Citrate Malate

Calcium citrate malate is a newly available form of calcium that is often added to orange juice and other beverages. It is highly absorbable and was the form of calcium used in many of the most positive studies of calcium and osteoporosis.

Tricalcium Phosphate

This form of calcium is also used to "fortify" foods and beverages and is fairly absorbable.

Safety Issues

In general, a daily intake of calcium up to 2,000 mg is safe, although there is no reason to take more than 1,200 mg.[13] However, if you have cancer, hyperparathyroidism, or sarcoidosis, you should take calcium only under the supervision of a physician.

Those with kidney stones or a history of kidney stones are often cautioned not to take supplemental calcium. The reason for this warning is that kidney stones are commonly made of calcium oxalate crystals. Yet recent studies have found that higher calcium intake does not increase the occurrence of kidney stones, and may even reduce it.[14] Nonetheless, if you have a tendency to form kidney stones, don't take high doses of calcium except on the advice of a physician.

Vitamin D is definitely safe when taken at 400 IU daily but can be toxic when taken at doses higher than 1,000 IU daily. This is because it's fat-soluble and can accumulate in the body. Toxicity symptoms caused by excess vitamin D include diarrhea, headaches, nausea, internal calcium deposits, and kidney stones. Those with sarcoidosis or hyperparathyroidism should definitely not take vitamin D except on medical advice.

Magnesium: Possibly Helpful for Osteoporosis

Magnesium is another mineral your body needs for its basic cellular functions and it, like calcium, is stored in the bones. In fact, about 60% of the body's total magnesium can be found in the skeleton. Magnesium appears to play an important role in protecting bone mass as well.

No large-scale studies have been conducted to determine whether supplemental magnesium helps to prevent osteoporosis. However, there is indirect evidence to support this theory: Women with osteoporosis have been shown to have lower-than-normal levels of magnesium in their bones. Magnesium may also play a role in producing activated vitamin D, which, as you've seen, helps maintain bone mass.

Foods rich in magnesium include wheat bran, almonds, cashews, blackstrap molasses, soybeans, tofu, collard greens, and avocado. The usual recommended dose for all women is 250 to 350 mg per day, but some alternative practitioners recommend more—400 to 800 mg per day—for menopausal women.[15] Magnesium is available in many different supplemental forms, all of which the body absorbs equally well.

When taken appropriately, magnesium is safe. However, people with severe kidney or heart disease should take it only under medical supervision.

Boron: Possibly Helpful for Osteoporosis but May Present Risks

Boron is a trace mineral that may help our bodies retain calcium levels. It is found in fruits and vegetables, and we probably get enough of it in our diet. Boron was once thought not to be important to human health. My college nutrition textbook, published in 1988, does not even mention it. However, some researchers now think that it may be important for postmenopausal women's health.

Based on a single study involving 12 postmenopausal women, it is suspected that boron may reduce the amount of calcium lost in the urine, potentially indicating a helpful effect on bone.[16] While the number of women in this study was much too small to draw any firm conclusions, based on its preliminary findings, many alternative practitioners now recommend boron as a supplement. However, more research is needed to substantiate its use.

Furthermore, this study raised a potential concern: Researchers also found that boron could raise the body's level of estradiol. Could this mean that it might also increase a woman's risk for developing estrogen-dependent cancers? Since you're most likely get all the boron your body needs from your diet, it's probably best not to take a boron supplement until more conclusive information is available on its risks and benefits. However, if you are interested in supplemental boron, there are many forms available in health-food stores and pharmacies.

The current prevailing wisdom is that a daily dosage of 1.5 to 3 mg is safe. The United States Department of Agriculture (USDA) has not established a recommended daily allowance for boron.

Vitamin E:
Reduces the Risk of Heart Disease

Vitamin E has long been considered likely to help relieve hot flashes and vaginal dryness. Even conventional physicians sometimes recommend it for this purpose. However,

there is little to no real evidence that it is effective for this purpose. But there is good evidence that vitamin E can reduce the risk of heart disease, a major concern for women in menopausal years and beyond.

The best study of vitamin E's effects on heart disease was a double-blind placebo-controlled trial of 2,002 individuals with proven coronary artery disease, 546 were given 800 IU of vitamin E daily, 489 were given 400 IU daily, and 967 were given a placebo.[17] Participants were fol-

Vitamin E is an antioxidant that appears to help protect the body against heart disease, cancer, and other illnesses.

lowed for an average of about 18 months. The treated individuals showed a significant drop in heart attacks.

Also, an observational study of 11,178 people aged 67 to 105 years found that those participants who were taking vitamin E supplements at the beginning of the study were found to have a 34% reduced likelihood of death from heart disease over the many years that the study continued.[18] Vitamin C supplements alone did not seem to make a difference, but the combination of vitamin E and C produced a 53% reduction in risk. Continued long-term use of vitamin E reduced the risk by 63%.

Finally, an 8-year study of 87,245 female nurses aged 34 to 59 with no previously diagnosed heart disease found that women who took vitamin E supplements for at least 2 years had a 40% reduced risk of developing coronary disease.[19] Consumption of other antioxidants such as vitamin C and beta carotene was not associated with much risk reduction.

Supplementation with B vitamins—specifically vitamin B$_6$ and folic acid—may also diminish your risk of heart disease.

Practitioners who recommend vitamin E supplements for menopausal women usually suggest a dosage of 400 to 800 IU a day.[20] This is much more than can possibly be obtained from food, so supplements are necessary.

Vitamin E is considered safe when used at this dosage, but it should not be combined with blood-thinning drugs such as Coumadin (warfarin), heparin, Trental (pentoxifylline), or aspirin. It also may be advisable not to combine vitamin E with natural substances that possess a mild blood-thinning effect, such as the herbs garlic and ginkgo.

B Vitamins:
May Also Help Prevent Heart Disease

Supplementation with B vitamins—specifically vitamin B$_6$ and folic acid—may also diminish your risk of heart disease.

You need to make sure you get enough vitamin B_{12} as well to properly utilize these vitamins.

According to the Nurses' Health Study, an enormous observational study of 121,700 female nurses that began in 1976, women with the highest intake of folic acid had half the risk of heart disease compared to those with the lowest intake.[21] Furthermore, each 100 mcg/day increase in intake lowered the risk by 5.8%. Positive results were also seen with vitamin B_6 intake.

In addition, women who got enough folic acid and vitamin B_6 were significantly less likely to suffer heart attacks compared to those who got much lower amounts. Researchers concluded that a higher intake of folic acid, either alone or in combination with vitamin B_6, significantly reduces the risk of heart disease and heart attack in women.

Dosage

The adult recommended daily value for folic acid is 400 mcg.[22] Since only about 10% of the people in the United States alone get 400 mcg daily, this vitamin is certainly worth paying attention to.[23]

Food sources, in order of higher to lower folic acid content, include brewer's yeast, black-eyed peas, soy flour, wheat germ, beef liver, soybeans, wheat bran, kidney beans, lima beans, asparagus, lentils, walnuts, fresh spinach, peanut butter, broccoli, whole wheat cereal, brussels sprouts, almonds, oatmeal, cabbage, avocado, green beans, corn, pecans, blackberries, and oranges.

The recommended daily value for vitamin B_6 is 2 mg for most adult men and 1.6 mg for most adult women.[24] Most multivitamin supplements contain at least 2 mg. In the studies described earlier, a 3 mg daily dose was found to be heart-protective. For those with heart disease, 4 mg daily has been suggested.

The average diet provides slightly less than the recommended daily value of this vitamin. Foods rich in vitamin

B_6 include meats, cereals, lentils, nuts, and certain fruits and vegetables, such as bananas, avocados, and potatoes.

The adult recommended daily value for vitamin B_{12} is 6 mcg. Meat, fish, eggs, and milk products provide plenty of vitamin B_{12}. However, among people of retirement age and older, deficiency does occur.[25,26] In particular, people with reduced levels of stomach acid (such as those taking ulcer medication) may not absorb B_{12} well from foods. The stomach acid is needed to separate B_{12} from protein. Fortunately, vitamin B_{12} taken in supplement form does not present this problem.

Clinical studies conducted in China suggest that gamma-oryzanol may help reduce menopause-related symptoms.

Safety Issues

Folic acid presents little risk of toxicity. It is water soluble and is rapidly eliminated from the body.[27]

Warning: You should not take more than 800 mcg of folic acid daily without a doctor's evaluation, not because it is toxic at that dose, but because it may mask the signs of vitamin B_{12} deficiency while irreversible nerve damage progresses.

Vitamin B_6 can be toxic at excessive doses, causing harm to the nerves. Such symptoms have appeared in doses as low as 150 mg, although they usually do not appear until you consume 500 mg a day or more for quite a long time.

Also, vitamin B_6 can work against the therapeutic effect of levodopa by preventing its active form from reaching the brain, so if you take levodopa (e.g., for Parkinson's disease), you should avoid vitamin B_6 supplements. This is probably not a problem with Sinemet (levodopa combined

Too Many Pills?

In chapter 3 we noted that one of the disadvantages of hormone-replacement therapy is that it commits you to taking a pill every day for the rest of your life. Vitamins and minerals also have an alarming way of adding up to a lot of pills, and they can be costly—I know people who spend between $50 and $400 each month on supplements! Fortunately, there are many good multivitamins with minerals. Taking one of these, and supplementing it if you need to, is probably the least expensive way to add vitamins and minerals to your diet, as well as the most convenient. For example, if you're concerned about osteoporosis and your multivitamin doesn't have the recommended dose of calcium, simply add a calcium supplement that brings the total daily amount of supplemental calcium to between 1,000 and 1,500 mg.

Many companies manufacture multivitamins that are specially designed for menopausal women. One of these may meet your needs better than most multivitamins. Because literally hundreds of vitamin products are available, you should shop around and consult your health-care practitioner to find one that suits you best.

with carbidopa), but you should check with your doctor to be safe.

Vitamin B_{12} appears to be essentially nontoxic, even in very high doses.

Gamma-Oryzanol: More Research Needed

Gamma-oryzanol (also known as ferulic acid), a substance made from rice bran, is widely touted as a treatment for menopausal symptoms. Preliminary clinical studies conducted in China support this contention.[28] However, further research is needed to truly document this potential benefit.

No significant side effects from gamma-oryzanol have been noted in clinical trials, but full safety studies have not been performed. The recommended dosage is 100 mg 3 times daily.

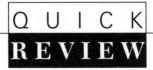

QUICK REVIEW

- Calcium alone, or, even better, calcium plus vitamin D can help prevent osteoporosis. Even if you are taking estrogen, calcium can provide additional benefit.

- Appropriate dietary intake of calcium is as follows: 400 mg daily for infants; 800 mg daily for children up to the age of 19; 1,000 mg daily for adults up to the age 50; and 1,200 mg per day for adults over 50 as well as for pregnant or nursing women.

- The usual recommendation for vitamin D is 400 IU daily. However, some studies cited used doses as high as 800 or 1,000 IU daily. Such doses should be taken only with medical supervision.

- Good food sources of calcium include dairy products and calcium-fortified orange juice, soy milk, and tofu.

- Calcium supplements made with oyster shells, dolomite, and bonemeal are inexpensive but may contain lead. Calcium carbonate is inexpensive and convenient but may not be absorbed well. Calcium citrate is easier to absorb but it's more expensive and you have to take more pills. Calcium citrate malate is also well absorbed, but it is most commonly found in beverages rather than in pill form.

- Taking various trace minerals (zinc, 15 mg; copper, 2.5 mg; and manganese, 5 mg) along with calcium and vitamin D may add additional benefit for osteoporosis prevention.

- Magnesium and boron have been proposed for osteoporosis, but they have not been proven effective, and there may be safety concerns with boron.

- Vitamin E and gamma-oryzanol are widely believed to reduce menopausal symptoms, but there is little documentation as yet that they are effective.

- Good evidence tells us that vitamin E can reduce the risk of heart disease. The usual dose is 400 to 800 IU daily. Do not combine high-dose vitamin E with blood-thinning drugs or herbs, such as Coumadin (warfarin), heparin, Trental (pentoxifylline), aspirin, garlic, or ginkgo, except on the advice of a physician.

- B vitamins such as B_6, folic acid, and B_{12} appear to lower the risk of heart disease. The recommended daily doses are: folic acid, 400 mcg; vitamin B_6, 4 mg; and vitamin B_{12}, 6 mcg (or more).

Lifestyle Changes

I n previous chapters I discussed the benefits and risks of various herbal and dietary treatments for the symptoms of menopause, as well as the long-term health risks that postmenopausal women face. You can enhance such treatments by looking at your life as a whole and making lifestyle changes to support good health. Diet, exercise, and your emotional life all play an important role in your health during and after menopause.

Furthermore, lifestyle improvements offer other benefits unmatched by any pill. After Mary Jo started HRT, she began to exercise several days a week and eat more carefully. As she explained, "I know I'm protecting my bones and my heart," she says, " but it's more than that. Taking care of myself this way makes me feel better today. Diet and exercise are the only medicines I know about that actually make you feel great every way at once."

She has a good point. Taking a calcium pill may make your bones stronger, but it doesn't change your whole day. Exercise and healthful eating habits are powerful preventive medicines against osteoporosis, heart disease, and cancer, and they provide benefits you can feel all over.

Foods to Include in Your Diet

Adding certain foods to your diet can improve your overall health and well-being. As many great healers have said, "Let food be your medicine." The following section will explain how certain foods can help maintain your health and also help alleviate menopausal symptoms.

Legumes (Beans)

You'll recall from chapter 8 that legumes such as soybeans and soy-based products contain isoflavones, which are a kind of phytoestrogen: a substance that has a weak estrogen-like effect in your body. Eating these foods can help reduce menopause-related symptoms and may also help prevent cardiovascular disease. Isoflavones are also present to some extent in other legumes, such as chickpeas (garbanzo beans), lentils, kidney beans, and black beans.

As many great healers have said, "Let food be your medicine."

Legumes are also a great source of protein, especially when combined with whole grains such as rice or barley. They are an excellent source of fiber as well, and contain many other nutrients such as calcium, magnesium, potassium, iron, and B vitamins. Because soy is very rich in isoflavones, it is particularly good for women during and after menopause, and it comes in so many forms—soy flour, soy milk, soy flakes, tofu, tempeh, soy cheese, even soy hot dogs—that it is easy to incorporate into your diet.

However, some people are allergic to soy. They may wish to increase their intake of other legumes instead.

Whole Grains

Whole grains such as oats, corn, barley, millet, buckwheat, and brown rice contain lignans, another type of phyto-estrogen. The richest source of lignans, however, is flaxseed, which also provides many essential fatty acids. Whole grains are high in fiber, carbohydrates, vitamins B and E, magnesium, calcium, and potassium as well.

Vegetables

Your grandmother was right when she told you to "eat your vegetables." We now know that a diet high in vegetables (and fruits) can dramatically reduce your odds of developing heart disease and cancer. Vegetables are rich in many vitamins, minerals, and fiber, including natural substances known as carotenes, all of which can give your body important support as you undergo the changes and stress of menopause. Dark green and yellow/orange vegetables are some of the best, but they are all good for you. Eat as great a variety as you can. The best way is to prepare them fresh and don't overcook them. Steaming is one of the most healthful methods. Collapsible stainless steel steamers that fit inside most saucepans are inexpensive and easy to find.

The richest source of lignans is flaxseed, which also provides many essential fatty acids.

Some wild plants are the most nutritious of all. I love going out in the springtime and collecting fresh dandelion leaves from my yard. The greens are usually not too bitter if you pick them before they flower. I usually steam them lightly and add a little lemon juice for a delicious addition to my meal.

Dandelions get a bad rap from lawn owners, but herbalists treat them with more respect. There is even a society in Cleveland, Ohio, called Defenders of the Dandelion, which promotes the many beneficial uses of dandelions and sponsors an annual National Dandelion Cook-Off. Dandelion is a good source of calcium, iron, magnesium, and other nutrients. Other nutritious wild plants include lamb's quarters, nettles, and wild asparagus. Homegrown vegetables are also healthful because nutrients don't have a chance to die on the long trip from field to market. They taste better, too.

Vegetables are rich in many vitamins, minerals, and fiber, including natural substances known as carotenes, all of which can give your body important support as you undergo the changes and stress of menopause.

Fruits

Along with vegetables, fruits can reduce your risk of developing cancer and heart disease. They are great sources of bioflavonoids, vitamin C, enzymes, and fiber. Fruits contain many other vitamins and minerals as well. They are best eaten fresh and whole, rather than made into juice. Fruit juices are usually very high in natural sugar, and they often lack some of the bioflavonoids that are found in the whole fruit. Juices also lack the fiber that is found in whole fruits.

If you like fruit drinks but want to gain the full nutritional benefit of whole fruit, try fruit smoothies. My friend Renee makes one every morning. She puts a frozen banana, some berries, and a little soy milk into a blender and purees it for a healthful drink.

Foods to Limit in the Diet

As we saw in chapter 2, certain foods and beverages may have a negative impact on your health if you consume large amounts of them. For example, soft drinks are high in phosphorus, which may increase postmenopausal health risks. The caffeine in black tea and coffee may also be harmful, although this is controversial, and some studies suggest that black tea and coffee may even offer some healthful benefits.

Along with vegetables, fruits can reduce your risk of developing cancer and heart disease.

Besides its other harmful effects, alcohol can intensify hot flashes. Most women can tolerate alcohol in moderation, and two drinks a day may be healthful, but excessive drinking could significantly worsen your symptoms as well as increase the risk of many diseases. You should also limit the amount of saturated fats in your diet. As we saw previously, saturated fats greatly increase cholesterol levels in your blood, which can lead to cardiovascular disease. The typical American diet, which contains excessive amounts of saturated fats, is thought to be largely responsible for the high incidence of cardiovascular disease and cancer in the United States.[1]

According to the American Heart Association, your total fat intake should be less than 30% of all your dietary calories, and your saturated fat intake should be less than

10%. One of the best ways to reduce your level of saturated fats is to limit your intake of red meat, dairy products, and saturated vegetable oils such as coconut and palm oil. You can substitute more plant-based protein from legumes and whole grains to improve your health. Replace your hamburger with a soy burger. Try lentil soup sometimes, instead of the usual beef noodle. You don't have to completely cut red meat and dairy from your diet, but ideally you should try to eat them only

Besides its other harmful effects, alcohol can intensify hot flashes.

once in a while rather than every day. Also, olive oil and canola oil are more healthful than butter or margarine.

Exercise

In many areas of our health, the benefits of consistent exercise are unparalleled. There simply is no substitute. Exercise is known to support the cardiovascular system, reduce blood sugar levels, promote strength and endurance, increase lung capacity, help with weight management, and balance your mental and emotional well-being.

Exercising also appears to be powerful medicine to prevent and even reverse bone loss and osteoporosis. Physically active people have higher bone densities than do otherwise similar individuals who are not active.[2] The peak bone mass of physically active women as they enter menopause is considerably higher than that of women of the same age with a sedentary lifestyle.

Indeed, physical inactivity is one of the known risk factors for osteoporosis. The doubling rate of hip fractures in the last 30 years is thought to be partly due to the drastic decrease in physical activity.[3] One of the most serious forms of inactivity is bed rest. It is known that total bed rest leads to a rapid and severe demineralization of bone, with a reduction in bone mass of about 1% per week![4] Thus physical activity truly plays a vital role in maintaining bone mass.

> **It is known that total bed rest leads to a rapid and severe demineralization of bone, with a reduction in bone mass of about 1% per week!**

Just as inactivity increases bone loss, exercise appears to stimulate bone growth. Heavy exercises such as running or playing ball games twice a week for 1 hour were found to result in an increase of 3.5% in bone mineral content after 8 months.[5] Jogging, rowing, and stair climbing has been found to produce a 5.2% increase in bone mineral content in the lower back after 9 months.[6] If intense physical activity is continued, there can be a total reversal of postmenopausal bone loss in the lower back.[7]

Indirect Benefits of Exercise

Exercise can also help osteoporosis indirectly. By increasing your strength and improving your balance, it makes you less likely to fall down and break your hip.

Exercise is also helpful if you already have broken a hip. However, it often happens that people who have broken a hip may be hesitant to walk or to try an exercise routine afterward for fear of falling again. Their self-confidence and trust in their balance may be diminished. While understandable, this reluctance can lead to a sedentary lifestyle and accelerated osteoporosis. If you are recovering from a hip fracture, seek proper physical therapy and guidance, so you can regain balance and stamina and prevent further bone loss.

Gloria's Story

Consider Gloria, a 72-year-old woman who was showering one morning when the phone rang. She rushed out of the shower to answer the phone, slipped on the wet floor, and broke her hip. She recovered fully but was left with a psychological scar: She was terrified to walk. Her fear kept her from regular activities. Gloria was afraid that she might lose her balance and fall again, so when she did walk, she had an unsure gait and touched the wall for support. With a lot of coaching, Gloria went to a class for stretching and strengthening. She was finally able to regain her balance and confidence.

What Is the Best Type of Exercise?

The choice of exactly which exercises are appropriate for you must be made on an individual basis, perhaps with the support of a professional sports medicine doctor, physical therapist, or physical trainer. We know that it is important to engage in activity that will hold your interest since consistency is a factor in increasing bone density.

For the purpose of combating osteoporosis, it appears that weight-bearing exercises such as walking, jogging, and stair climbing may be best. They generate a mechanical stress to the bones that sends signals to the body to produce new bone.

There are many conflicting ideas about how much exercise we need. A reasonable recommendation is 20 minutes a day, 5 days a week; or 1 hour a day, 3 days a week.

To create an exercise program for yourself, you don't necessarily have to join a gym. Although many women like them—gyms have all the equipment and support you will need—others find them intimidating, and not everyone can afford the membership fees.

The best way to exercise is to get your body moving by doing something you truly take pleasure in. Are you partial to walking, biking, hiking, dancing, tennis, basketball, or jogging? The important thing is to find something you enjoy enough to do regularly. Personally, I like to dance. Early in the morning, I warm up with some slow music. After a few songs I switch to rock and roll for a fun aerobic workout. This type of exercise works for me because it expresses who I am, letting me combine my love of music and the joy of dance to feed my body both physically and emotionally. Because I enjoy it so much, it becomes a playful activity, not a "workout," so I exercise more often than I would if I considered it a chore.

Just as inactivity increases bone loss, exercise appears to stimulate bone growth.

Walking is another form of exercise that can be pleasurable, especially if you make into a social event. When I lived near my sisters, we often walked to the local reservoir. Not only could I give them regular botany lessons in the process, but it allowed us to spend time together. This is why many women form walking groups, to combine regular physical exercise with the added benefit of social contact and emotional support. A group can also give you friendly encouragement to exercise when you might otherwise skip a day. There are days when I'm not in the mood or feel I don't have the time, but then a friend calls me up, and off I go!

Stress Reduction

Change itself is stressful, and because of this, menopause can be a very tense time. Along with the hormonal changes of menopause, a woman often finds herself dealing with anxiety-producing events such as the death or illness of aging parents. Her children may be leaving home just as her parents begin to need her more. We can't always avoid these situations, but we can change the way we deal with them. Dietary changes can help us cope. Exercise, especially yoga, can provide emotional as well as physical support. When I feel stressed out, I usually go for a brisk walk. Connecting with nature gives me strength and energy, so I always feel much better after trekking up one of the mountains near my home.

Yoga is an ancient tradition whose practitioners believe it can improve your nervous, endocrine, and digestive systems.

Relaxing exercises such as yoga can also help. Yoga is a form of meditative exercise that greatly increases your flexibility through a series of stretching postures. It's a great way to reduce stress and tension, too; its benefits are both physical and emotional.

Yoga is an ancient tradition whose practitioners believe it can improve your nervous, endocrine, and digestive systems. There have been no scientific studies to prove or disprove these claims, but yoga's popularity as a means to improve health and reduce tension has been rising steadily for two decades.

Many people achieve excellent results with yoga. If you have never tried it before, you should consider taking a beginners' class where you can learn to do the postures safely. Yoga has become so popular that it isn't difficult to find classes, which can cost from $10 to $20 for a 2-hour class. Many adult education programs offer yoga classes. There are also numerous excellent books and videos available.

My friend Margaret recently bought a yoga videotape and now does yoga every morning. She says that adding it to her daily routine has helped her to feel more emotionally centered. However, yoga is best learned from a teacher who can watch you and let you know if you are doing the postures correctly.

Keep in mind that if you're thinking of making significant lifestyle changes, you should take it slowly. Make small changes one at a time, rather than attempting too many changes at all once. Above all, have fun and relax. Avoid being too rigid about your diet or exercise regimen.

The lifestyle changes mentioned in this chapter are meant to help you feel better, so only do what you feel comfortable doing. What works for one person might not work for you. Experiment until you find a balance that suits you.

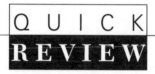

QUICK REVIEW

- A diet low in saturated fats and high in whole grains, fresh fruits, and vegetables can reduce your chances of developing cancer and heart disease.

- Regular exercise can actually reverse osteoporosis.

- There are many conflicting ideas about how much exercise we need. A reasonable recommendation is 20 minutes a day, 5 days a week; or 1 hour a day, 3 days a week.

- Stress-reducing activities can go a long way toward keeping you healthy and happy, during and after menopause.

Acupuncture and Chinese Herbal Medicine

I n this book, I have described several herbal and dietary methods that you can use to reduce the symptoms and long-term risks of menopause. Many of these have a reasonably sound scientific basis and can be used with confidence of success. However, there is another approach that is widely used for women going through menopause: acupuncture and Chinese herbal medicine. Although these traditional Chinese treatments have little valid scientific evidence supporting them, I will briefly discuss them because they are so widely believed to be effective.

Acupuncture and Chinese Herbology

Acupuncture is a centuries-old therapy that originated in China and established itself in Japan, Korea, and other Asian nations. It involves the insertion of thin needles just beneath a person's skin. Acupuncture is traditionally combined with a complicated system of herbal medicine known simply as Chinese herbal medicine. Together, these are the most well-known and widely accepted forms of traditional Chinese medicine. Practitioners of various types of alternative medicine believe that these Chinese approaches are particularly successful at treating the symptoms of menopause, including hot flashes, mood swings, and anxiety.[1] However, there's no real scientific evidence to cite in proof of their effectiveness.

> **Chinese medicine is passionately holistic in nature. This means that practitioners take into account all of a person's physical, emotional, and mental symptoms, viewing the many seemingly unrelated parts as one single unified "pattern."**

Traditional Chinese medicine is more than 3,000 years old and is based on a much different view of the human body than is found in Western medicine. Chinese medicine is passionately holistic in nature. This means that practitioners take into account all of a person's physical, emotional, and mental symptoms, viewing the many seemingly unrelated parts as one single unified "pattern." For example, the following symptoms would be considered unrelated to each other in Western medicine: a feeling of heat, anger bubbling just below the surface, headaches, cramps and digestive problems, cysts, and insomnia. Yet any practitioner of Chinese medicine would immediately draw them all together into a single "pattern" with the poetic name "congested liver energy." Treatment would be based on taking care of this underlying problem, rather than addressing each condition singly.

Along with Chinese herbs, acupuncture is primarily a way of working with patterns of illness in Chinese medicine. Acupuncture works with *meridians,* a system of "energy channels" that are thought to pervade the body. According to Chinese medicine, life-force energy called *qi* (pronounced "chee") flows along these meridians. The theory is that if the *qi* does not flow properly, disease can result. Instead of treating the disease per se, Chinese medical treatment aims to improve and balance this "energy flow."

In acupuncture, needles are placed under the skin at specific points along the meridians. There are 361 acupuncture points in the body. A typical treatment will target several points along one or more meridians. Typically, 4 to 12 needles are used in a single treatment. Today, all practitioners use disposable needles to eliminate the risk of blood-borne diseases. Chinese herbal treatment typically accompanies acupuncture.

One of the most commonly asked questions about acupuncture is, "Does it hurt?" Actually there is little or no pain involved in a typical acupuncture treatment. The needles are very thin, much thinner than those doctors use to give injections. Most of the time, the person scarcely feels the needle going in. Occasionally there is a dull, mild aching sensation at the site of the needle, and occasionally a needle will draw a tiny amount of blood or leave a small bruise. Serious complications are rare, but occasionally an incautious acupuncturist can puncture the lung or a large

In Chinese medicine, the body is seen as an integrated system of energy channels called *meridians.* According to the theory of Chinese medicine, life-force energy called *qi* flows along these meridians.

blood vessel. However, acupuncturists are specially trained to minimize the possibility of either of these complications. In fact, acupuncturists receive years of training, and many states require them to be licensed or registered. A qualified acupuncturist can answer any questions you might have about safety.

Acupuncture is regarded as a gradual therapy that takes time, but it is believed by its practitioners to produce results that persist even after treatment is stopped. On the down side, there is little scientific evidence that acupuncture is effective, the skill level of acupuncturists varies widely, and it is an expensive approach to health care.

Finding an Acupuncturist

Acupuncture is a legally authorized form of health care in more than 30 states. As mentioned previously, many of these states require acupuncturists to be licensed. There is also a National Commission for the Certification of Acupuncture and Oriental Medicine, whose Web site includes a directory of acupuncturists who have passed their stringent qualifying exam. The address to their Web site is www.nccaom.com (see the appendix for the organization's full mailing address).

It is worth taking care in choosing a practitioner. Look for someone who is willing to spend time with you on your initial visit. Before recommending treatment, a good acupuncturist will ask you detailed questions about your health and symptoms and

Contrary to popular fears, acupuncture rarely hurts. The needles used in acupuncture are much thinner than needles used to give injections. Most people don't even feel them.

Can Acupuncture
Help Menopausal Symptoms?

Cynthia McMahon King, a licensed acupuncturist, pharmacist, and homeopath from Boxborough, Massachusetts, uses both acupuncture and Chinese herbs in the treatment of menopausal women. Cynthia says, "I see a lot of menopausal women with hot flashes, loss of libido, and heavy bleeding. I feel very confident in offering treatment to these women because so many women have had excellent results. One of my patients came in experiencing loss of libido. Her husband was very much against her seeing an acupuncturist; he thought it was all a scam. After a few weeks of treatment, she felt a lot better, and her husband became a believer!" Of course, anecdotes like this don't prove anything. Properly performed studies must be conducted, and so far all of the well-designed studies of acupuncture have been too small to prove anything conclusively.

will also give you a brief physical examination (disrobing is not necessary). This examination usually begins with the acupuncturist taking your pulse by placing the index, middle, and ring fingers for a rather long time on first one wrist and then the other. This is classic Chinese *pulse diagnosis*. Then the acupuncturist will examine your tongue and/or gently probe your abdomen for tender spots to diagnose your condition and decide how to treat it. An acupuncturist who simply hears your story and starts putting in needles is not practicing the traditional art.

I received acupuncture for 1 year for the treatment of mid-cycle bleeding. My gynecologist determined that the bleeding resulted from a hormone imbalance and wanted me to start taking birth control pills. This didn't feel right to me, so I went to another doctor who was willing to work with my acupuncturist and me. I saw positive results within the first 3 weeks. After about 8 months of treatment, my cycles were completely back to normal.

Generally, about six sessions of acupuncture will give you an indication of whether the treatment is going to work for you. If you find some relief in this time period, you may wish to stay with the treatment. If you haven't experienced any effects within 6 weeks, you'll have to decide whether to continue with a few additional acupuncture sessions or try another form of treatment instead.

Chinese Herbalists

Chinese herbology operates according to the same theory as traditional Chinese acupuncture, but it uses herbs rather than needles to restore energy balance. Like an acupuncturist, a Chinese herbalist will begin by asking you a number of specific questions about your health and symptoms. As with acupuncture, each herbal treatment is individually tailored. Chinese herbalists prescribe specific combinations of many herbs, usually to be taken in the form of a tea, but possibly as a capsule or tablet. Practitioners usually recommend that the herbs be taken two to four times a day for a period of one to several months— so be prepared to work these into your daily schedule.

Acupuncture is a legally authorized form of health care in more than 30 states, and many of these states require acupuncturists to be licensed.

Herbal medicine is frequently combined with acupuncture, but not all acupuncturists are well-versed in Chinese herbal medicine. In general, at least 500 hours of extra study are required to attain a basic level of proficiency in Chinese herbal medicine.

Many herbal stores sell prepackaged, standard Chinese herbal formulas in capsule form, but these products aren't a good substitute for seeing a qualified herbalist. For one thing, the standard formulas aren't likely to meet your needs as well as a specially prescribed formula will. Another factor to consider is that your needs may change over time, as you respond to the treatment. Your herbalist will adjust your formula as needed. You can find a list of licensed Chinese herbalists on the Web site for the National Commission for the Certification of Acupuncture and Oriental Medicine.

As with acupuncture, each herbal treatment is individually tailored. Chinese herbalists prescribe specific combinations of many herbs, usually to be taken in the form of a tea, but possibly as a capsule or tablet.

There is one issue with Chinese herbal medicine that I should mention, however: safety. Virtually all Chinese herbs are grown in China under unknown quality-control conditions. Concerns have been raised about possible contamination with pesticides and, in the case of prepackaged formulas, also heavy metals, and Western drugs. The fundamental safety of many of the herbs themselves and the complex combinations in which they are prescribed have not been scientifically established either.

Cost

Acupuncture can be a fairly expensive form of treatment because it's so labor-intensive. One session can cost from

$45 to $100. Since a typical course of treatment requires a weekly session for at least 10 weeks, and weekly treatment for a year or more is common, the overall costs can be high. Furthermore, Chinese herbs can cost an additional $20 to $100 per month. Some insurance plans cover acupuncture and even Chinese herbology, but many do not.

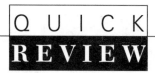

- Acupuncture and Chinese herbology are the two best-known and most widely accepted forms of traditional Chinese medicine.
- Although there has been little scientific evaluation of these ancient arts, they are widely believed to be quite effective at treating menopausal symptoms.
- Acupuncture and Chinese herbology can be used separately, although they are most often used together.
- A typical course of acupuncture involves the insertion of 4 to 12 long, thin needles into specific points along one or more of the body's meridians.
- Acupuncture is a time-consuming and relatively expensive form of treatment, but if it works for you, its benefits are said to last long after the period of treatment. An acupuncture treatment typically costs from $45 to $100 and a typical course of treatment involves a weekly session for 10 or more weeks.
- Chinese herbs are widely regarded as quite potent, but there are safety concerns regarding them.
- A course of herbal treatment typically lasts from one to several months and can cost from $20 to $100 per month.

Putting It All Together

For your easy reference, this chapter contains a brief summary of key information contained in this book. Please refer to earlier chapters for more comprehensive informtion, including a detailed discussion of safety issues.

Today, a woman entering menopause has many different options for treating her symptoms, if they occur, and for protecting her long-term health. Each woman must ask herself a number of questions: Should I replace my hormones by taking medication? Do I want to take medications for the rest of my life? If I choose natural alternatives, which ones are the most reliable and effective? How great is my risk for osteoporosis and heart disease?

In this book, I have given you some information about many of the available treatments. This final chapter will provide examples of how these treatments can be combined with dietary and lifestyle changes to create a personalized holistic regimen. Here are two different scenarios, each showing a possible treatment regimen for a menopausal woman. These scenarios are some of the many possible ways that a woman could combine the available options. I offer them to give you ideas for developing your own treatment regimen, based on your doctor's advice as well as your personal goals, philosophy, and needs. A full discussion of safety issues and other considerations may be found in the appropriate chapters.

Scenario #1:
Conventional Hormone Treatment

If you opt for conventional hormone-replacement therapy (HRT), your heath-care provider will help you decide which is the best treatment protocol for you. New drugs such as raloxifene give you more options than ever to receive benefits while reducing risks.

In addition to hormone therapy, you can also help maintain your health by making certain dietary and lifestyle changes. For example, you may want to add a **calcium** supplement and **vitamin D** to your diet to help prevent bone loss. Clinical studies have shown that using calcium in addition to HRT preserves bone density more effectively than using HRT alone. To help protect yourself against osteoporosis, you should take between 1,000 and 1,200 mg of calcium per day, combined with vitamin D at a dose of 400 IU daily.

Adding **magnesium** (250 to 350 mg daily), **zinc** (15 mg), **copper** (1 to 3 mg), and **manganese** (5 mg) may provide further benefit. **Boron** is another potentially important mineral, although there are some safety concerns about its use. If you suffer from serious kidney or heart disease, consult a physician before taking any of these supplements.

To help reduce your risk of cardiovascular disease, you should cut the amount of saturated fats in your diet. The best way to decrease some of these "bad" fats is to limit red meat, dairy products, and coconut and palm oils. Add plenty of whole grains, beans, fish, vegetables, and fruit to your diet to help keep your body strong and healthy. **Vitamin B$_6$** (a minimum of 3 mg daily) and **folic acid** (400 mcg daily) may help reduce homocysteine levels, further protecting your heart. **Vitamin E** (400 IU daily) will add antioxidant protection.

Finally, you can add regular aerobic and weight-bearing exercise to your routine. Consistent exercise will help protect you against osteoporosis and cardiovascular disease. Take a walk during your lunch hour. This not only helps to strengthen your body, but it can also release any stress that has built up during your workday.

Scenario #2: All-Natural Treatment

If you prefer not to use hormones during menopause, there are herbs, vitamins, minerals, and dietary and lifestyle changes you can use to reduce menopausal symptoms and help prevent osteoporosis and cardiovascular disease. However, keep in mind that none have been proven as effective as estrogen for preventing cardiovascular disease and osteoporosis.

There is some scientific evidence that the herb **black cohosh** can considerably reduce most menopausal symptoms, including hot flashes, vaginal dryness, and anxiety. The usual daily dose of black cohosh is 1 to 2 tablets (2 mg each) of 27-deoxyacteine twice daily. However, we don't know whether it reduces the risk of osteoporosis or cardiovascular disease. Although black cohosh appears to be safe in general, we don't know whether it is okay for women who have already had breast cancer to take it.

Two small double-blind studies suggest that the herb **kava** can specifically reduce the anxiety and depression associated with menopause. **Garlic** may reduce the risk of heart disease, and **St. John's wort** may alleviate depression.

Phytoestrogens such as those found in **soy** can help lessen your menopausal symptoms. Soy can also protect your cardiovascular system by reducing the cholesterol in your bloodstream and may help prevent breast and other hormone-sensitive cancers. As little as 25 g of soy protein daily should be enough to produce positive effects.

The phytoestrogen **ipriflavone** has been found to slow or even reverse osteoporosis. The proper dose of ipriflavone is 200 mg 3 times daily or 300 mg 2 times daily. Although ipriflavone is not believed to increase the risk of cancer, as with black cohosh, women who have already had breast cancer should use ipriflavone only on the advice of a physician.

All the dietary, lifestyle, and vitamin and mineral suggestions made in the first scenario apply here as well: adequate amounts of **calcium, vitamin D, magnesium, manganese, zinc, copper, vitamin B$_6$, folic acid,** and **vitamin E;** as well as fruits and vegetables; a lowfat diet; and regular exercise.

If you are not using conventional hormone treatment, it is especially important to have a bone density screening done to get a base level reading of your bone strength. This test should be redone periodically to determine whether additional treatment is necessary.

These choices can be confusing. It might help to remember that, above all, you should feel comfortable with the regimen you decide upon. You have the right to choose a mode of treatment that is compatible with your philosophy and your values. For most women, there isn't a single best approach. It is also possible to change your mind after starting one type of treatment if you find that it isn't working. Discovering the best treatment for yourself might be a process of trial and error, combined with research and close consultation with your physician.

Appendix

Referrals

American Association of Naturopathic Physicians
601 Valley Street
Seattle, Washington 98109
Phone: (206) 298-0125
Web site for referrals: www.naturopathic.org

**American Holistic Medical Association and
  American Holistic Nurses Association**
4101 Lake Boone Trail, Suite 201
Raleigh, NC 27607
  Referrals: Written requests only. Send $8.00 for a directory of members; all members are M.D.s, D.O.s (osteopaths) or R.N.s

**National Certification Commission for Acupuncture
  and Oriental Medicine**
11 Canal Center Plaza
Alexandria, VA 22314
Phone: (703) 548-9008
Web site for referrals: www.nccaom.org

Organizations

North American Menopause Society
Post Office Box 94527
Cleveland, OH 44106
Phone: (216) 844-8748
Web site: www.menopause.org

National Women's Health Network
514 10th Street, NW, Suite 400
Washington, DC 20004
Phone: (202) 347-1140

National Osteoporosis Foundation
1150 17th Street NW, Suite 500
Washington, DC 20036
Phone: (202) 223-2226
Web site: www.nof.org

American Heart Association
7320 Grenville Avenue
Dallas, TX 75231
Phone: (214) 373-6300
Web site: www.amhrt.org

Organizations for Herbal Information

Herb Research Foundation
1007 Pearl Street, Suite 200
Boulder, CO 80302
Phone: (303) 449-2265
Web site: www.herbs.org

The Herb Research Foundation (HRF) is a nonprofit organization that provides accurate and biased information on the health benefits of plants. HRF offers custom research on herbs, spices, and medicinal plants for a nominal fee. They also offer over 150 informational packets that provide the consumer with a thorough introduction to many common herbs and health condi-

tions. Membership includes a complementary copy of
HerbalGram or Herbs for Health Magazine, a quarterly
newsletter, and discounts for all informational services.

American Botanical Council

Post Office Box 210660
Austin TX 78720-1660
Phone: (512) 331-8868
Web site: www.herbalgram.org

The American Botanical Council is a nonprofit organization whose main goal is to educate the public about the benefits of herbs and plants. Together with the Herb Research Foundation, they publish the journal *HerbalGram,* an outstanding magazine that provides information on botanical research, conferences, legal issues, and market reports. They have an extensive bookstore, which carries numerous books on herbs, including hard to find European books on herbal medicine.

American Herbal Pharmacopoeia

Post Office Box 5159
Santa Cruz, CA 95063
Web site: www.herbal-ahp.org

The American Herbal Pharmacopoeia is a nonprofit organization dedicated to the development of herbal monographs containing accurate, critically reviewed information on botanicals to provide guidance in the appropriate use of herbal therapeutics. These monographs provide detailed descriptions of each herbs history, botany, pharmacognosy, chemistry, analytical methods, and clinical therapeutics.

Support Groups
Self-Help Clearinghouse
St. Clares-Riverside Medical Center
25 Pocono Road
Denville, NJ 07834
Phone: (201) 625-7101
> This group has information about support groups for
> various illnesses.

Recommended Reading
Menopause/Women's Health
Gretchen Henkel. *The Menopause Source Book.* Lowell
    House Books; Los Angeles. 1998
Christiane Northrup. *Women's Bodies, Women's Wisdom:
    Creating Physical and Emotional Health and Healing.*
    Bantam Books; New York. 1994
Susun S. Weed. *Menopausal Years: The Wise Women
    Way.* Ash Tree Publishing; Woodstock, New York. 1992
Susan Love, M.D. *Dr. Susan Love's Hormone Book.* Ran-
    dom House; New York. 1997
Susan M. Lark, M.D. *The Estrogen Decision: A Self Help
    Book.* Celestial Arts; Berkeley, California. 1995
Nina Shandler. *Estrogen The Natural Way: Over 250
    Easy and Delicious Recipes for Menopause.* Villard
    Books; New York. 1997

Women's Herbals
Rosemary Gladstar. *Herbal Healing For Women.* Simon
    and Schuster; New York. 1993
Amanda McQuade Crawford. *The Herbal Menopause
    Book: Herbs, Nutrition, and Other Natural Therapies.*
    The Crossing Press; Freedom, California. 1996
Deb Soule. *The Roots of Healing: A Women's Book of
    Herbs.* Citadel Press Book; Secaucus, New Jersey. 1995

Amanda McQuade Crawford. *Herbal Remedies For Women.* Prima Publishing; Rocklin, California. 1997

Other Books

Michael T. Murray. *Encyclopedia of Nutritional Supplements.* Prima Publishing; Rocklin, California. 1996

Michael Murray, N.D. and Joseph Pizzorno, N.D. *Encyclopedia of Natural Medicine. Revised 2nd Edition.* Prima Publishing; Rocklin, California. 1998

Notes

Chapter One

1. Kim JG, et al. Autoimmune premature ovarian failure. *J Obstet Gynaecol* 21: 59–56, 1995.

2. Martin E. Medical metaphors of women's bodies: menstruation and menopause. *Int J Health Serv* 18: 237–254, 1988.

3. Barbre JW. Meno-boomers and moral guardians: an exploration of the cultural construction of menopause. Menopause: a midlife passage. Indiana University Press: Indianapolis, 1993.

4. Weed SS. Menopausal years: the wise woman way. Woodstock, New York.: Ash Tree Publishing, 1992.

5. Lock M. Menopause in cultural context. *Experimental Gerontology* 29: 307–317, 1994.

6. Lock M. Contested meanings of the menopause. *The Lancet* 337: 1270–1272, 1991.

7. Martin MC, et al. Menopause without symptoms: the endocrinology of menopause among rural Mayan Indians. *Am J Obstet Gynecol* 168: 1839–1843, 1993.

8. Northrup C. Women's bodies, women's wisdom. New York: Bantam Books, 1994.

9. Lark SM. The estrogen decision: self help book. Berkeley, California: Celestial Arts, 1995.

10. Shaw CR. The perimenopausal hot flash: epidemiology, physiology, and treatment. *Nurse Pract* 22: 55–56, 1997.

11. Lark SM. 1995.

12. Love SM. Dr. Susan Love's hormone book: making informed choices about menopause. New York: Random House, 1997.

Chapter Two

1. Lindsay R. Osteoporosis: a guide to diagnosis, prevention, and treatment. National Osteoporosis Foundation. New York: Raven Press, 1992.

2. Osteoporosis. National Institute of Health Consensus Development Statement. April 2–4; 5(3), 1–6, 1984.

3. Northrup C. Menopause. *Primary Care: Clinics in Office Practice* 24(4): 921–948, 1997.

4. Luckey MM, et al. A prospective study of bone loss in African-American and white women: a clinical research center study. *Journal of Clinical Endocrinology and Metabolism* 81(8): 2948–2956, 1996.

5. Bowmen MA and Spangler JG. Osteoporosis in women. *Primary Care: Clinics in Office Practice* 24(1): 27–36, 1997.

6. Sharp PC and Kunen JC. Women's cardiovascular health. *Primary Care: Clinics in Office Practice* 24(1): 1–14, 1997.

7. Schaefer EJ, et al. Lipoprotein (a) levels and risk of coronary heart disease in men: the lipid research clinics coronary primary prevention trial. *JAMA* 271: 999–1003, 1994.

8. Love SM. Dr. Susan Love's hormone book. New York: Random House, 1997.

9. American Heart Association, American Cancer Society. Living well, staying well. New York: Times Books and Random House, 1996: 11.

Chapter Three

1. Wilson R. Feminine forever. New York: Evans, 1966.

2. Hemminki E and Sinikka S. A review of postmenopausal hormone replacement therapy recommendations: potential for selection bias. *Obstetrics and Gynecology* 82(6): 1021–1028, 1993.

3. Colditz GA, et. al. The use of estrogens and progestins and the risk of breast cancer in postmenopausal women. *NEJM* 332: 1589–1593.

4. Grodstein F, Stampfer M, Manson J, et al. Postmenopausal estrogen and progestin use and the risk of cardiovascular disease. *N Engl J Med* 335: 453–460, 1996.

5. Sharp PC and Kunen JC. Women's cardiovascular health. *Primary Care: Clinics in Office Practice* 24(1): 1–14, 1997.

6. Knopp PH, et al. Effects of estrogens and lipoprotein metabolism and cardiovascular disease in women. *Atherosclerosis* 110(suppl): S83, 1994.

7. Schaefer EJ, et al. 1994. Lipoprotein (a) levels and risk of coronary heart disease in men: the lipid research clinics coronary primary prevention trial. *JAMA* 271: 999–1003, 1994.

8. Sotelo MM and Johnson SR. The effects of hormone replacement therapy on coronary heart disease. *Endocrinology and Metabolism Clinics* 26(2): 313–328, 1997.

9. Hulley S, et al. Randomized trial of estrogen plus progestin for secondary prevention of coronary heart disease in postmenopausal women. *Journal of the American Medical Association* 280: 605–613, 1998.

10. Ettinger R, et al. Long term estrogen replacement therapy prevents bone loss and fractures. *Ann Intern Med* 102(3): 319–324, 1985.

11. Cauley JA, et al. Estrogen replacement therapy and fractures in older women: study of osteoporotic fractures research group. *Ann Intern Med* 122(1): 9–16, 1995.

12. Marcus R. for the PEPI Trial Investigators: Effects of hormone replacement therapies on BMD: results from the postmenopausal estrogen/progestin intervention trial. *J Bone Miner Res* 10(suppl.1): 276, 1995.

13. Love SM. Dr. Susan Love's hormone book. New York: Random-House, 1997.

14. Bryant HU and Dere WH. Selective estrogen receptor modulators: an alternative to hormone replacement therapy. *Proc Soc Exp Biol Med* 217(1), 45–52, 1998.

15. Bryant HU and Dere WH. 1998.

16. Sadovsky Y. Editorials. Selective modulation of estrogen receptor action. *Journal Clinical Endocrinology and Metabolism* 83(1): 31–35. 1998.

17. Bryant HU and Dere WH. 1998.

18. Johnson SR. Menopause and hormone replacement therapy. *Medical Clinics of North America* 82(2): 297–320, 1998.

19. Lippman M, et al. Effects of estrone, estradiol and estriol on hormone-responsive human breast cancer in long-term tissue culture. *Cancer Research* 37:1901–1907, 1977.

20. Love SM. 1977

21. Lark SM. The estrogen decision: self help book. Berkeley, California: Celestial Arts, 1995.

22. Lark SM. 1995.

23. Hudson T. Townsend Letters for Doctors and Patients. Port Townsend, WA, 1996, Issue No. 156.

24. Lee J. Osteoporosis reversal, the role of progesterone. *International Nutrition Review* 10 (3): 384–391, 1990.

25. Grady D, et al. Hormone therapy to prevent disease and prolong life in postmenopausal women. *Ann Inter Med* 117: 1016–1037, 1992.

26. Brinton LA, et al. Menopausal estrogens and breast cancer risk: An expanded case-control study. *Br J Cancer* 54(5): 825–832, 1986.

27. Brinton LA. Hormone replacement therapy and risk for breast cancer. *Endocrinology and Metabolism Clinics* 26(2): 361–378, 1997.

28. Writing Group for the PEPI Trial. Effects of hormone replacement therapy on endometrial histology in postmenopausal women: The postmenopausal estrogen/progestin intervention trial. *JAMA* 275(5): 370–375, 1996.

29. Johnson SR. 1998.

Chapter Four

1. Samuelsson G. Drugs of natural origin: a textbook of pharmacognosy. Sweden: Swedish Pharmaceutical Press, 1992.

Chapter Five

1. Stolze H. An alternative to treat menopausal complaints. *Gyne* 3: 14–16, 1982.

2. Warnecke G. Influencing menopausal symptoms with a phytotherapeutic agent. *Med Welt* 36: 871–874, 1985.

3. Duker DM, et al. Effects of extracts from *Cimicifuga racemosa* on gonadotropin release in menopausal women and ovariectomized rats. *Planta Medica* 57(5):420–424, 1991.

4. Jarry H, et al. Endocrine effects of constituents of *Cimicifuga racemosa*. The effect on serum levels of pituitary hormones in ovariectomized rats. *Planta Med* 1: 46–49, 1985a.

5. Stoll W. Phytopharmacon influences atrophic vaginal epithelium. Double-blind study: *Cimicifuga* vs estrogenic substances. *Therapeuticum* 1: 23–31, 1987.

6. Schaper & Brümmer. Remifemin®: a plant-based gynecological agent. Scientific brochure, 1997.

7. Schulz V. Rational phytotherapy. New York: Springer, 1998.

8. Korn WD. Six month oral toxicity study with remifemin-granulate in rats followed by an 8-week recovery period. Hanover, Germany: International Bioresearch. 1991.

9. Liske E. Therapeutic efficacy and safety of *Cimicifuga racemosa* for gynecological dsorders. *Advances in Therapy* 15: 45–53, 1998.

10. Nesselhut T, et al. Influence of *Cimicifuga racemosa* extracts with estrogen-like activity on the vitro proliferation of mamma carcinoma cells. *Arch Gynecol Obstet* 254: 817–818, 1993.

Chapter Six

1. Volz HP, et al. Kava-kava extract WS 1490 versus placebo in anxiety disorders—a randomized placebo-controlled 25 week outpatient trial. *Pharmacopsychiatry* 30(1): 1–5, 1997.

2. Warnecke G. Neurovegetative dystonia in the female climacteric. Studies on the clinical efficacy and tolerance of kava extract WS-1490. *Fortschr Med* 109:119–122, 1991.

3. Warnecke G, et al. Wirksamkeit von Kawa-kawa-extract beim klimakterischen Syndrom. *Z Phytother* 11: 81–86, 1990. [Cited in Shulz, V. et al Rational phytotherapy, New York: Springer-Verlag, 1998.]

4. Jussofie A., et al. Kavapyrone enriched extract from *Piper methysticum* as modulator of the GABA binding site in dif-

ferent regions of rat brain. *Psychopharmacology,* 116: 469–474, 1994.

5. Munte TF, et al. Effects of oxazepam and an extract of kava roots *(Piper methysticum)* on event-related potentials in a word recognition test. *Neurophychobiology* 27(1): 46–53, 1993.

6. Heinze HJ, et al. Pharmacopsychological effects of exazepam and kava-extract in a visual search paradigm assessed with event-related potentials. *Pharmacophychiatry* 27(6): 224–230, 1994.

7. Herberg KW. Effect of kava-special extract WS 1490 combined with ethyl alcohol on safety-relevant performance parameters. *Blutalkohol* 30(2): 96–105, 1993.

8. Schulz V, et al. Rational phytotherapy. New York: Springer-Verlag, 1998: 72.

9. Duffield PH and Jamieson D. Development of tolerance to kava in mice. *Clinical and Experimental Pharmacology and Physiology* 18: 571–578, 1991.

Chapter Seven

1. Ernst E. St. John's wort, an anti-depressant? A systematic, criteria-based review, *Phytomedicine* 2(1): 67–71, 1995.

2. Laakman, G, et al. St. John's wort in mild to moderate depression: The relevance of hyperforin for the clinical efficacy. *Pharmacopsychiatry* 31(suppl): 54–9, 1998.

3. Hänsgen KD, et al. Multicenter double blind study examining the antidepressant effectiveness of the *Hypericum* extract LI 160. *Journal of Geriatric Psychiatry and Neurology* 7: S15–S18, 1994.

4. Harrer G and Sommer H. Treatment of mild/moderate depressions with *Hypericum. Phytomedicine* 1: 3–8, 1994.

5. Vorbach EU, et al. Therapy for insomniacs. Effectiveness and tolerance of valerian preparations. *Psychopharmakotherapie* 3:109–115, 1996.

6. Holzl J, et al. Receptor binding studies with *Valeriana officinalis* on the benzodiazepine receptor. *Planta Med* 55: 642, 1989.

7. Schulz V, et al. Rational phytotherapy. New York: Springer-Verlag, 1998: 72.

8. Albrecht M, et al. Psychopharmaceuticals and safety in traffic. *Z Allg Med* 71: 1215–1221, 1995.

9. Gerhard U, et al. Vigilance-decreasing effects of 2 plant-derived sedatives. *Schweiz Rundsch Med Prax* 85(15): 473–481, 1996.

10. Silagy CA, et al. A meta-analysis of the effect of garlic on blood pressure. *J Hypertens* 12(4): 463–468, 1994.

11. Warshafsky S, et al. Effect of garlic on total serum cholesterol. A meta-analysis. *Ann Intern Med* 119(7, Part 1): 599–605, 1993.

12. Mader FH. Treatment of hyperlipidaemia with garlic-powder tablets. Evidence from the German Association of General Practitioners' multicentric placebo-controlled double-blind study. *Arzneimittelforschung* 40(10): 1111–1116, 1990.

13. Neil HA, et al. Garlic powder in the treatment of medoerate hyperlipidaemai: a controlled study and meta-analysis. *J R Coll Physicians Lond* 30(4): 329–334, 1996.

14. Simons LA, et al. On the effect of garlic on plasma lipids and lipoproteins in mild hypercholesterolaemia. *Atherosclerosis* 113(2): 219–225, 1995.

15. Santos OA de A, et al. Effects of garlic powder and garlic oil preparations on blood lipids, blood pressure and well being. *Br J Clin Res* 6: 91–100, 1995.

16. Silagy CA, et al. A meta-analysis of the effect of garlic on blood pressure. *J Hypertens* 12(4): 463–468, 1994.

17. Schulz V, et al. Rational phytotherapy. New York: Springer-Verlag, 1998.

18. Breithaupt-Grogler K, et al. Protective effect of chronic garlic intake on the elastic properties of the aorta in the elderly. *Circulation* 96(7): 2649–2655, 1997.

19. Schulz V, et al. 1998.

20. Hirata JD, et al. Does dong quai have estrogenic effects in postmenopausal women? A placebo-controlled trial. *Fertil Steril* 68 (6): 981–986, 1997.

Chapter Eight

1. Adlercreutz H and Mazur W. Phyto-oestrogens and western disease. *Annals of Medicine* 29: 95–120, 1997.

2. Aldercreutz H. Evolution, nutrition, intestinal microflora, and prevention of cancer: A hypothesis. *Proc Soc Exp Biol Med* 217(3): 241–246, 1998.

3. Adlercreutz H and Mazur W. 1997.

4. Murkies AL, et al. Clinical review 92: Phytoestrogens. *J Clin Endocrin Metab* 83(2): 297–303, 1998.

5. Murkies AL, et al. Dietary flour supplementation decreases post-menopausal hot flashes: effect of soy and wheat. *Maturitas* 21(3): 189–195, 1995.

6. Albertazzi P, et al. The effect of dietary soy supplementation on hot flashes. *Obstst Gynecol* 91(1): 6–11, 1998.

7. Kurzer MS and Xu X. Dietary phytoestrogens. *Ann Rev Nutr* 17: 353–381, 1997.

8. Kurzer MS and Xu X. 1997.

9. Anderson JW, et al. Meta-analysis of the effects of soy protein intake on serum lipids. *New England Journal of Medicine* 333(5): 276–282, 1995.

10. Baum J, et al. Long-term intake of soy protein improves blood lipid profiles and increases mononuclear cell low-density-lipoprotein receptor messenger RNA in hypercholesterolemic, postmenopausal women. *Am J Clin Nutr* 68: 545–51, 1998.

11. Genari C, Adami S, Agnusdei L, et al. Effect of chronic treatment with ipriflavone in postmenopausal women with low bone mass. *Calcif Tissue Int* 61: S19–S22, 1997.

12. Valente M, Bufalino L, et al. Effects of 1-year treatment with ipriflavone on bone in postmenopausal women with low bone mass. *Calcif Tissue Int* 54: 377–380, 1994.

13. Kovacs AB. Efficacy of ipriflavone in the prevention and treatment of postmenopausal osteoporosis. *Agents Actions* 41: 86–87, 1994.

14. Adami S, et al. Ipriflavone prevents radial bone loss in postmenopausal women with low bone mass over 2 years. *Osteoporos Int* 7(2): 119–125, 1997.

15. Agnusdei D, et al. Efficacy of ipriflavone in established osteoporosis and long-term safety. *Calcif Tissue Int* 61(1): S23–27, 1997.

16 Kovacs AB. Efficacy of ipriflavone in the prevention and treatment of postmenopausal osteoporosis. *Agents Actions* 41: 86–87, 1994.

17. Agnusdei D, Camporeale F, et al. Effects of ipriflavone on bone mass and bone remodeling in patients with established postmenopausal osteoporosis. *Curr Ther Res* 51(1): 82–1, 1992.

18. Melis GB and Paoletti AM. Ipriflavone and low doses of estrogens in the prevention of bone mineral loss in climacterium. *Bone and Mineral* 19: S49–56, 1992.

18. Nozaki M, Hashimoto K, et al. Treatment of bone loss in oophorectomized women with a combination of ipriflavone and conjugated equine estrogen. *Int J Gyn Ob* 62: 69–75, 1998.

19. Adlercreutz H and Mazur W. 1997.

20. Adlercreutz H. Phytoestrogens: epidemiology and a possible role in cancer prevention. *Environ Health Perspect* 103 (suppl 7): 103–112, 1995.

21. Lee HP, et al. Dietary effects on breast-cancer risk in Singapore. *Lancet* 337: 1197–1200, 1991.

22. Ingram D, et al. Case-control study of phyto-oestrogen and breast cancer. *Lancet* 350: 990–994, 1997.

Chapter Nine

1. Reid IR. The roles of calcium and vitamin D in the prevention of osteoporosis. *Endocrinol Metab Clin North Am* 27: 389–398, 1998.

2. Cumming RG. Calcium intake and bone mass: A qualitative review of the evidence. *Calcif Tissue Int* 47: 194–201, 1990.

3. Dawson-Hughes B, Dallal GE, Krall EA, et al. A controlled trial of the effect of calcium supplementation on bone density in postmenopausal women. *N Engl J Med* 323(13): 878–883, 1990.

4. Prince R. Diet and the prevention of osteoporotic fractures. *N Eng J Med* 337(10): 701–702, 1997.

5. Dawson-Hughes B, Dallal GE, Krall, EA. The effect of vitamin D supplementation on wintertime and overall bone loss in healthy postmenopausal women. *Ann Intern Med* 115(7): 505–512, 1991.

6. Dawson-Hughes B, Harris S, Krall E, et al. Effect of calcium and vitamin D supplementation on bone density in men and women 65 years of age or older. *N Engl J Med* 337(10): 670–673, 1997.

7. Nnieves JW, Komar L, Cosman F, et al. Calcium potentiates the effect of estrogen an calcitonin on bone mass: Review and Analysis. *Am J Clin Nutr* 67(1): 18–24, 1998.

8. Aloia JF, et al. Calcium supplementation with and without hormone replacement therapy to prevent postmenopausal bone loss. *Annals Intern Med* 120: 97–103, 1994.

9. Lloyd T, Andon MB, Rollings N. Calcium supplementation and bone mineral density in adolescent girls. *J Am Med Assoc* 270(7): 841–844, 1993.

10. Saltman PD, et al. the role of trace minerals in osteoporosis. *J Am Coll Nutr* 12(4): 384–389, 1993.

11. Strause L, et al. Spinal bone loss in postmenopausal women supplemented with calcium and trace minerals. *J Nutr* 124:1060–1064, 1994.

12. Adapted from Gebhardt S, and Matthews R. Nutritive values of foods, U.S.D.A., 1981. Pennington, JAT and Church, HN. Food values of portions commonly used. New York: Harper and Row, 1985. Brown SE. Bones better body. New Caanan: Keats Publishing, Inc., 1996.

13. NIH Consensus Development Panel on Optimal Calcium Intake. Nutrition 11: 409–411, 1994.

14. Curhan GC, Willett WC, Rimm EB. Comparison of dietary calcium with supplemental calcium and other nutrients as factors affecting the risk of kidney stones in women. *Ann of Int Med* 126: 497–504, 1997.

15. Murray M and Pizzorno J. 1998.

16. Neilson FH, et al. Effect of dietary boron on mineral, estrogen, and testosterone metabolism in postmenopausal women. *Fed Am Soc Exp Biol* 1(5): 394–397, 1987.

17. Stephens NG, Parsons A, Schofield PM, et al. Randomized controlled trial of vitamin E in patients with coronary disease: Cambridge heart antioxidant study (CHAOS). *Lancet* 347: 781–786, 1996.

18. Losonczy KG, Harris TB, Havlik RJ. Vitamin E and vitamin C supplement use and risk of all-cause and coronary heart disease mortality in older persons: The established populations for epidemiologic studies of the elderly. *Am J Clin Nutr* 64: 190–196, 1996.

19. Stampfer M, Hennekens C, Manson J, et al. Vitamin E consumption and the risk of coronary heart disease in women. *N Engl J Med* 328: 1444–1449, 1993.

20. Murray M and Pizzorno J. Encyclopedia of natural medicine. 2nd edition. Rocklin, California: Prima Publishing, 1998.

21. Rimm EB, et al. Folate and vitamin B6 from diet and supplements in relation to risk of coronary heart disease among women. *JAMA* 279(5): 359–364, 1998.

22. Covington R, (Ed.) Handbook of nonprescription drugs. American Pharmaceutical Association, 1996.

23. Rimm EB, et al. Folate and vitamin B6 from diet and supplements in relation to risk of coronary heart disease among women. *JAMA* 279(5): 359–364, 1998.

24. Covington R, (Ed.) 1996.

25. Saltzman, JR. et al. Effect of hypochlorhydria due to omeprazole treatment or atrophic gastritis on protein-bound B12 absorption. *J Am Coll Nutr* 13(6): 584–91, 1994.

26. Van Goor et al. Review. Cobalamin deficiency and mental impairment in elderly people. *Age Aging* 24: 536–42, 1995.

27. Covington R, (Ed.) 1996.

28. Werbach MR. Nutritional influences on illness. 2nd edition. Tarzana, California: Third Line Press, 1996.

Chapter Ten

1. Aldercreutz H and Mazur W. Phytoestrogens and western diseases. *Annals of Medicine* 29: 95–120, 1997.

2. Dalen N, Bone mineral content and physical activity. *Acta Orthop Scand* 45: 170–174, 1974.

3. Law MR, et al. Strategies for prevention of osteoporosis and hip fractures. *Br Med J* 303: 453–459, 1991.

4. Ernst E. Can exercise prevent postmenopausal osteoporosis? *Br J Sp Med* 28(1): 5–6, 1994.

5. Krolner B, et al. Physical exercise as prophylaxis against involuntary vertebral bone loss: a controlled study. *Clin Sci* 64: 541–546, 1983.

6. Ayalon J, et al. Dynamic bone loading exercises for postmenopausal women. *Arch Phys Med Rehab* 68: 280–283, 1987.

7. Krolner B, et al.

Chapter Eleven

1. Bratman S. The alternative medicine ratings guide: an expert panel ranks the best treatments for over 80 conditions. Rocklin, CA: Prima Health, 1998.

Index

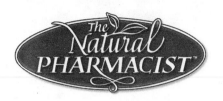

About the Author

Joanne Marie Snow is an herbalist, consultant, and botanical researcher with a bachelor's degree in biology. With more than 15 years in the health field, she has lectured at both national and international herbal symposiums, and has published several herbal monographs. She lives in Rutland, Massachusetts.

About the Series Editors

Steven Bratman, M.D., medical director of Prima Health, has many years of experience in the alternative medicine field. A graduate of the University of California at Davis, Medical School, he has also trained in herbology, nutrition, Chinese medicine, and other alternative therapies, and has worked closely with a wide variety of alternative practitioners. He is the author of *The Natural Pharmacist: Your Complete Guide to Herbs* (Prima), *The Natural Pharmacist: Your Complete Guide to Illnesses and Their Natural Remedies* (Prima), *The Natural Pharmacist Guide to St. John's Wort and Depression* (Prima), *The Alternative Medicine Ratings Guide* (Prima), and *The Alternative Medicine Sourcebook* (Lowell House).

David J. Kroll, Ph.D., is a professor of pharmacology and toxicology at the University of Colorado School of Pharmacy and a consultant for pharmacists, physicians, and alternative practitioners on the indications and cautions for herbal medicine use. A graduate of both the University of Florida and the Philadelphia College of Pharmacy and Science, Dr. Kroll has lectured widely and has published articles in a number of medical journals, abstracts, and newsletters.